D0094965

Making Soaps
& Scents

Making Soaps
& Scents

PERFUMES, SOAPS, SPLASHES & SHAMPOOS
THAT YOU CAN MAKE AT HOME

By Catherine Bardey

Photographs by Zeva Oelbaum

**BLACK DOG
& LEVENTHAL
PUBLISHERS**
NEW YORK

Copyright © 1999
Black Dog & Leventhal Publishers, Inc.

All rights reserved. No part of this book may be reproduced in
any form or by any electronic or mechanical means, including
information storage and retrieval systems without written
permission of the publisher.

Published by
Black Dog & Leventhal Publishers, Inc.
151 West 19th Street
New York, NY 10011

Distributed by Workman Publishing Company
708 Broadway
New York, NY 10003

Manufactured in the United States of America

ISBN 1-57912-059-8
h g f e

Library of Congress Cataloging-in-Publication Data

Bardey, Catherine, 1963-
Making Soaps & Scents/ by Catherine Bardey.
p.   cm.
Includes bibliographical references and index.
ISBN 1-57912-059-8
1. Soap 2. Perfumes. I. Title. II. Title: Making soaps and scents.
TP991.B27 1999   99-40548
668'.54--dc21   CIP

Design by 27.12 design, Ltd.
Studio photographs by Zeva Oelbaum

Table of Contents

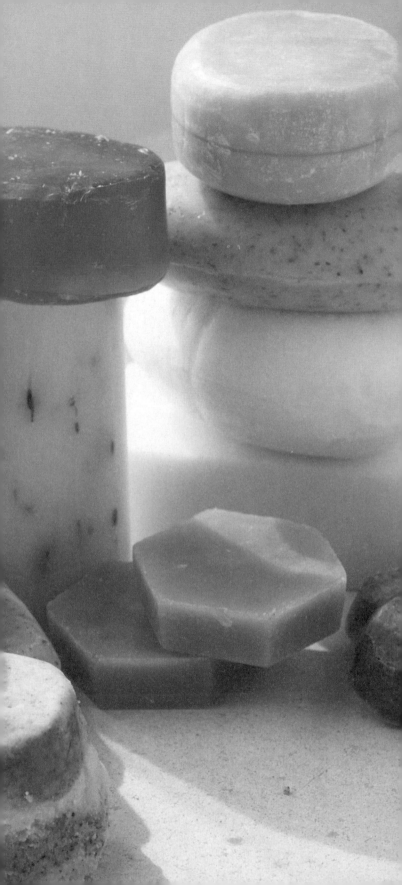

Making Soaps

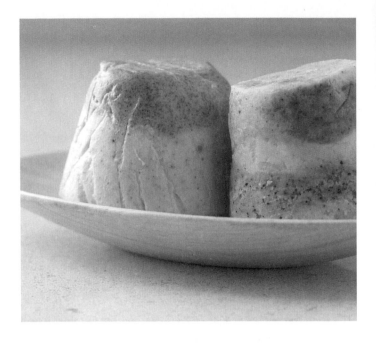

Soap has been around for a long time.

Not always in the shape of the Moisturizing Honey Almond Soap with Nutmeg or even the Cleansing Lavender Key Lime Soap flecked with purple petals and delicately scented with citrus aroma, mind you, but soap, a substance that lathers and cleans.

Legend has it that soap got its name from Mount Sapo, a hill in Rome on which animals were ritually sacrificed. At the bottom of the hill ran the Tiber River, where people would gather daily to wash their laundry. Rain would trickle down the hill into the river, carrying with it a clay-like substance of animal fats and wood ash residue from the sacrifices. Somehow, someone made the connection that the clay mixed in with the river's water produced a foamy substance that made the laundry cleaner.

Bathing was first popularized in Western culture by the famous Roman baths, the first of which was built in 312 bc. Soap, however, was not part of the bathing ritual and did not become analogous to personal hygiene until the second century. Prior to that, milk, sand, oils, herbs, flower petals and various ointments were the cleansing materials of choice. Rubbed on the body, they removed dirt, grime and dead skin cells. It's not until Galen of Pergamom (ca. 130-ca. 200), one of the most outstanding physicians of antiquity after Hypocrites, who recognized soap for its medicinal and cleansing properties, that the connection was made.

Unfortunately, after the fall of the Roman Empire and during the Dark Ages, bathing and basically any activities that focused on the human body became synonymous with evil doings. The concept of personal hygiene—and the use of soap specifically for that purpose—went into serious decline. As a result of the unsanitary living conditions, plague, disease and death became rampant throughout all of Europe.

Soap slowly began to re-emerge in certain parts of 8th century Italy and Spain, and later in 13th century France and then England. The advancements of a couple of very important French scientists in the 18th and 19th centuries further encouraged the fabrication and use of soap as a personal cleansing tool: Nicholas Leblanc patented a process in 1791 for making alkali (a necessary element in soap-making) from salt, and Louis Pasteur established the connection between bacteria and disease in the 1800s and hence the necessity to fight bacteria.

The advent of chemicals and the refinement of commercial soap-making methods have facilitated the production of long-lasting, rich-lathering soaps, and have made them an easy-to-obtain commodity. While the soap that we use today has undergone numerous transformations since the soap that our ancestors first lathered, the basic process of what soap is and what makes it work remains the same. This same, basic process can be reproduced in your home with a few simple ingredients and a couple of straightforward techniques.

Crafting customized soap is a truly rewarding pursuit. More and more people are rediscovering the pleasures of synthetic-free bubbles, and are exploring the creative depths behind fabricating a personalized bar. Whether it's Summer Citrus Soap, Chocolate Milk Soap or the more classic Coconut Rosewood bar that tickles your fancy, a little practice, patience and imagination will surely send you foaming!

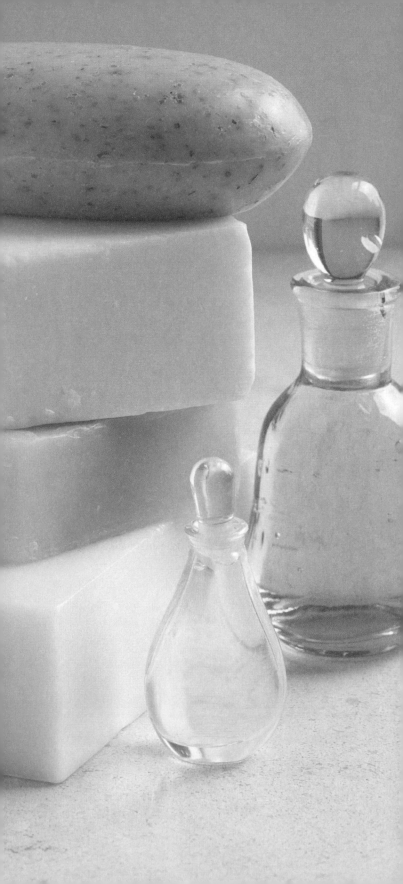

SOAP MAKING, IN A NUTSHELL

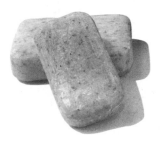

From raw ingredients to final form, all soap goes through a series of stages before it can be used. You can start from scratch and make cold process soap, or skip some steps and hand-mill or use the Jell-O method, but no matter which route you choose, all soap will have gone through all of these stages at some point. Basically, making soap involves the following:

• HEATING: two mixtures—one composed of oils, one of lye and water—are brought to a high temperature and combined.

• SAPONIFICATION: the chemical reaction between the oils, lye and water.

• MOLDING: liquid soap is poured into prepared molds, and set aside to dry and harden.

• SITTING, CURING and AGING: the process in which a batch of soap dries and cures, over a period of weeks.

Only after these four steps are completed is soap safe to use— but there are possibilities for adding your own personal touch all along the way, from what sort of oils you start with to moisturizing additives, fragrances, textures and colors.

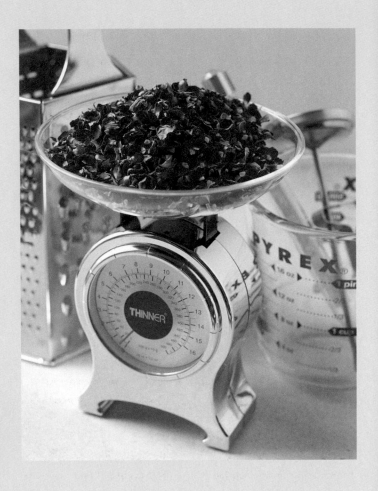

One of the pleasures of making your own soap is that you don't need any fancy or expensive equipment. In fact, most of the tools you'll be using can be found right in your own kitchen. From cheese graters to spatulas and hot mitts—and with a little imagination, confidence and creativity—you will be able to set up your workspace comfortably in no time at all.

- Scale: if you're going to be splurging on anything, this is probably where you should do it. The scale will be your most important tool. If you have or can get one that's electronic and digital, then you're way ahead of the game. An accurate measure of the ingredients—especially the lye solution, fats and oils—is crucial to soap making. Remember: weighing ingredients instead of measuring them by volume yields more precise results.

- Sharp paring knife for cutting, slicing and trimming bars of soap out of the slab and for scraping off excess soda ash.

- Measuring cups (glass) and spoons (stainless steel): to measure additives, softeners, essentials oils, herbs and spices, fruit or anything else that you will be adding to personalize your soap recipes.

- Large lye-resistant (stainless steel or ceramic) lobster/spaghetti pot : this is the master pot in which all the ingredients—fats or oils, lye/water solution and additives (softeners, scents, dyes)—will be blended. An eight quart-size pot will give you enough room.

- A two-quart lye-resistant container (glass or plastic) with a wide opening to pour out the lye/water solution into the master pot.

- Rubber or latex gloves: as a protective device, especially against lye, which will irritate and burn skin when in direct contact with it. Keep them on through the whole process, even when slicing and handling the hardened soap after it has cooled. The pH of the hardened soap is not fully established until the aging process is complete (see page 46 to learn more about the aging process).

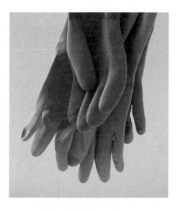

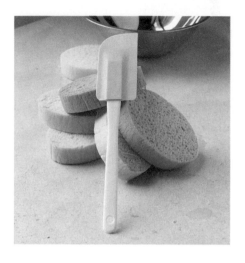

- Protective eye gear: a pair of glasses or goggles to protect your eyes from lye fumes, especially when the lye is mixed with the water, creating a vapor which can burn or sting the eyes.

- Disposable facemask (optional): available in hardware stores, a disposable facemask (the kind construction workers wear) helps minimize inhalation of noxious lye fumes.

- Cheese grater: for grating soap leftovers to make hand-milled soap(see page 50).

- Coffee grinder or food processor: for grinding herbs, spices, flowers, fruit, etc.

- Stainless steel large spoon for stirring and blending ingredients in the master pot.

- Stainless steel soup ladle: for ladling the liquid pre-set soap into small molds.

- 2 rubber or latex spatulas: for scraping liquid soap out of the master pot when pouring it into larger molds.

- 2 candy thermometers: these are crucial to getting the fats, oils, and lye solution at the right temperature. Stainless steel thermometers, preferably the kind that clip on to the side of the pot, give a more accurate reading.

- Old blankets or towels: for covering the soap for the

cooling and aging process (see page 46 for cooling and aging process).

- Stainless steel whisk (optional): for blending stubborn batches.

- Plastic wrap: to minimize soda ash or to use as a mold liner instead of vegetable spray.

- Wax paper (optional): can also be used as a mold liner. You'll need tape to secure the edges of the wax paper down on the outside of the mold.

- Hot mitts or pot holders.

- 2 water baths (optional): a bucket, large basin or sink in which to cool the lye/water solution, or to heat/cool oils.

- Sponges: it's good to have one of these handy in case there's a spill in the work area which calls for immediate clean-up.

- Various plastic, plastic-lined containers or heavy cardboard boxes and molds (see page 43 for molds).

- Non-stick vegetable spray or petroleum jelly: for greasing molds.

- Lye (flakes, beads, or granules): lye or sodium hydroxide can be purchased in hardware stores. It must be 100% pure sodium hydroxide.

- Water: distilled or right from the tap.

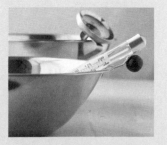

NOTE: *Glass, hard plastic, stainless steel, ovenproof stoneware or enamel are safe materials to use when making soap. Tin, aluminum, Teflon, zinc, copper and iron may corrode when in contact with lye. Avoid using anything made out of wood (spoons, spatulas); they are harder to clean and can splinter with age. Make sure you thoroughly clean all equipment after each use.*

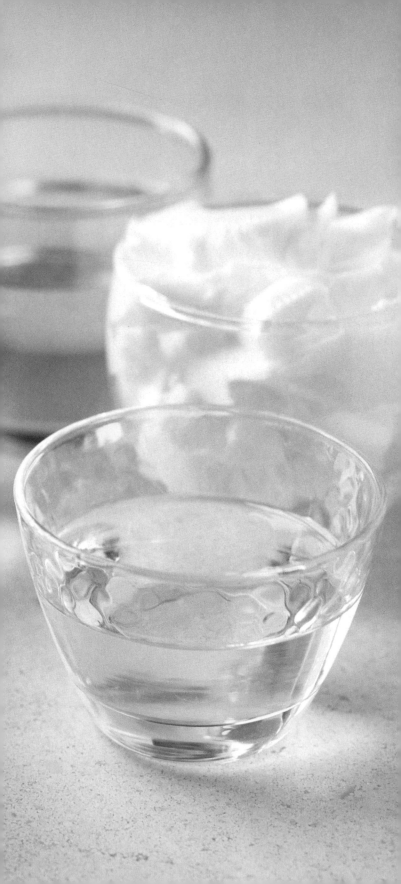

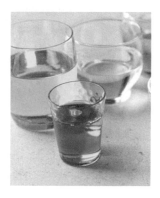

Soap is a combination of just a few simple ingredients: fats and/or oils, water and lye (sodium hydroxide). A dash of this or a smidgen of that can be added here or there to bring character to the bar like color, texture and skin softening qualities, but basically homemade soap is created out of the same stuff today as it was when it was first put to use.

Base Fats & Oils

Before getting set up to make your first batch, you will need to decide whether you want an animal fat based soap, a vegetable based one or a combination thereof. Each type of soap provides different properties and characteristics. What type of soap you choose to make will depend on your personal preference, on what supplies are readily available in your neighborhood and on what budget constraints you have.

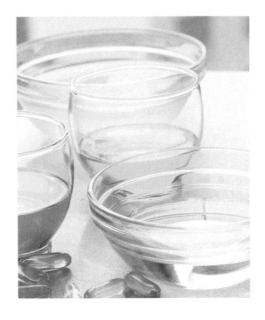

Vegetable-based soaps

V egetable-based soaps are softer than animal fat-based soaps, and therefore don't last as long. Conversely, their lather tends to be richer and smoother. One of the advantages of working with oils over animal fat is that there is no rendering process. Most—if not all—of the oils that you purchase on the market today are already purified and ready to use. The flip side is that vegetable oils can be more expensive than animal fats.

The oil you choose will depend on the quality and character you want to give the final product. Most manufacturers who make vegetable-base soap will select an oil for their base—such as coconut oil or palm oil—that is readily available and relatively inexpensive. Other oils, such as avocado oil, wheat germ oil or apricot oil (which are more expensive) are then added to the base to enhance the quality of the soap. The character, texture and properties of the final bar will depend on the types of oils and additives that were mixed in with the basic oil. Remember to check the saponification chart on page 170 to figure out how much lye you'll need to use for the oil that you have selected.

Types of basic oils & vegetable fats:

COCONUT OIL: This oil comes from the meat of the coconut and is available in most grocery stores, bakery stores, and specialty food shops. When you buy coconut oil, it can be either clear and liquid (if the room is warm enough) or thick and white (if the room is cooler), in which case it just needs to be heated up a bit to return to its liquid state. Coconut oil yields a creamy soap that is firm and lathers nicely. Its drawback is that it can dry out skin. To counteract this effect, moisturizing oils are often added to the coconut oil base.

COCOA BUTTER: Cocoa butter, obtained from the seeds of the cocoa tree, is a rich skin soother and softener that yields a creamy soap. It's available in candy-making supplied stores, health food stores and certain pharmacies.

OLIVE OIL: Olive oil is a known skin moisturizer that helps seal in the skin's natural moisture. There are many different grades of olive oil, with differences in color, aroma, flavor and price. Essentially, any grade of olive oil can be used for soapmaking. Extra-virgin and virgin olive oils, which come from the first cold pressing of the olives, are fragrant and deeply golden, and can leave your soap smelling like olives and looking a bit yellow. These oils also tend to take longer to saponify. Olive oil obtained from the last pressing of the olives (also called pomace oil) is practically odorless, a lot less expensive, and can saponify quickly. It yields a firm, high-quality soap with smooth—not abundant—lather.

PALM OIL: Palm oil is derived from the oil palm tree and its properties are very similar to that of tallow. Soap made from palm oil is easy to work with because it reacts predictably to the lye–water mixture and therefore saponifies well (see saponification process on page 34). Much like tallow, it yields a firm, longer lasting soap, but with a fairly weak lather. Palm oil, available in specialty food stores, is often used in conjunction with other oils that will enhance the quality of the lather without altering the beneficial properties of palm oil.

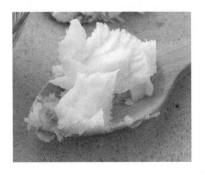

VEGETABLE SHORTENING: This thick white substance which looks like vanilla icing is primarily made out of soybean oil. It is best when used in conjunction with other oils and not as a main ingredient. It adds stability and bulk to the soap and blends well with other primary oils and additives.

Animal fat-based soaps

In the past, even homemade soap has been made from animal fat, primarily because it was readily available and inexpensive. Whether tallow, lard, beef fat or suet, there was always some form of fatty left-overs lying around the kitchen, and what better way to get rid of them and put them to good use than by making soap! Meat trimmings, cracklings and fat drippings were stored and accumulated and usually picked up by the local soapmaker in exchange for a couple of bars of soap to be delivered at a later date. The soapmaker would then melt down the fats and clean them in preparation for saponification

Today, many soap manufacturers continue to use animal fat. Tallow is the fat of choice because it is still less expensive and easier to process than most other fats or oils. Chances are the bar of soap on your local drugstore or supermarket's shelf is a tallow-based soap, with other ingredients—natural and synthetic—blended in for added richness and lather.

In general, animal fat-based soaps tend to be harder and last longer than their vegetable counterparts, thus making them more economical. The longer it lasts, the less often you need to buy it. Economics aside though, soap aficionados might argue that animal fat is the only way to go simply because, traditionally, that is how soap was made. They might also argue that animal fat is a more effective moisturizer than vegetable oil. It is true that certain vegetable oils, when over-applied, can sometimes dry out skin. On the other hand, there have been studies to suggest that due to the highly saturated nature of animal fat, it can clog pores and cause skin irritations on people with sensitive skin. Obviously, your own skin offers the best litmus.

The next thing to consider is lather and bubble quality. Some people like a soap that lathers abundantly; others prefer more discrete suds. Tallow, and animal fat in general, yields a mild and cleansing soap, but one that is not famous for the richness of its lather. In fact, soap manufacturers will add a vegetable oil—usually coconut—to the animal base to enhance the quality of the lather. But ultimately, if oodles of bubbles and foam are what you're after, than a vegetable-base soap is more likely up your alley.

Types of animal fat:

BEEF FAT AND SUET: Beef fat and suet (the fat that directly surrounds the cow's kidneys) are available from your local butcher or supermarket, and are inexpensive. The main difference between beef fat and suet is that suet tends to be firmer and cleaner than regular beef fat. But both beef fat and suet need to be rendered into tallow before use. Both yield a mild soap with a hard texture.

TALLOW: This is the ingredient of choice, simply because it is the purest and easiest to work with. Tallow is obtained through a process called rendering tallow. Essentially what this means is that beef fat or suet is cut into pieces, melted down in a big pot and then purified by straining the melted liquid several times to remove all impurities. Once cool, the final product is a firm, whitish substance with practically no smell. Rendering tallow is an extremely important step in the soap making process. All soapmakers will agree that the cleaner the tallow, the better the soap. If the fat is not properly cleansed, the soap might end up streaked, discolored or worse yet, have an unpleasant and rancid smell to it.

LARD: Lard is the same thing as tallow, except that the rendered fat is pig fat, not beef. Lard is inexpensive and can sometimes be found packaged and sold in supermarkets.

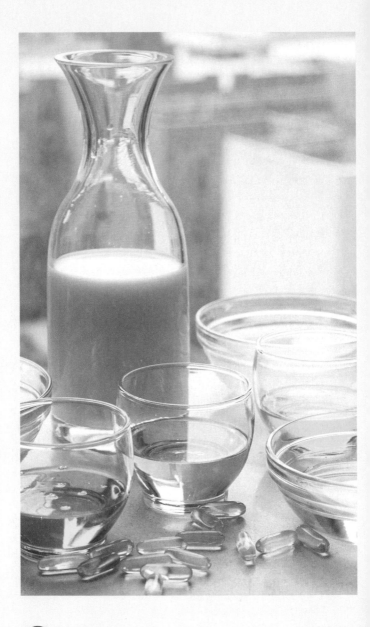

Once you have selected your base fats and/or oils, you can start customizing your soap by adding other ingredients—such as softeners, exfoliating agents and emollients—to the base. Remember to keep in mind that whatever oil you add to the base will affect the saponification process. Consult the saponification chart on page 167 to make the proper lye adjustments.

Skin Softeners, Moisturizers, & Emollients:

These additives will enhance the soap's moisturizing and soothing properties. Some of the ingredients (like jojoba and olive oil) act as barriers on the skin to seal in the skin's natural moisture and prevent moisture loss caused by the environment. Others, like avocado or sweet almond oil, contain certain components like vitamins, proteins and amino acids that actually have a healing and soothing effect on the skin.

ADDITIVE	HOW MUCH	WHEN TO ADD TO THE OIL/FAT BASE
aloe gel	1 tbls	• right before pouring in molds
apricot kernel oil	1 tbls	• right before pouring in molds
avocado oil	1 tbls	• right before pouring in molds
castor oil	1 tbls	• right before pouring in molds
honey	1 tbls	• right before pouring (warmed) in molds
karite butter (or shea butter)	1 tbls	(melted & cooled) • right before pouring in molds
carrot oil	3/4 tbls	• before adding lye/water mixture
jojoba oil	1 tbls	• right before pouring in molds
milk (butter milk, goat's milk, cow's milk, coconut milk or cream)	1/4 cup	• right before pouringin molds
powdered milk	1/8 cup	• right before pouring in molds
sweet almond oil	1 tbls	• right before pouringin molds
wheat germ oil	3/4 tbls	• before adding lye/water mixture

(table based on 3 lb. batch of soap)

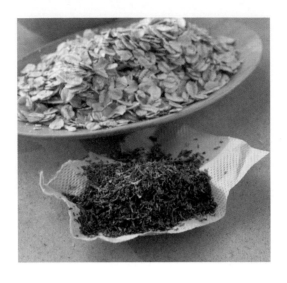

Exfoliants

Exfoliants act as abrasives and will help cleanse your skin by rubbing off the surface layer of dead skin cells. Before adding them to your soap batch, make sure the ingredients are ground finely enough. You don't want to feel as though you are rubbing your skin with sandpaper and you certainly don't want to risk clogging your drain.

ADDITIVE	HOW MUCH	WHEN TO ADD TO THE OIL/FAT BASE
Alfalfa meal	1/4 cup	• right before pouring in molds
Bran	1/4 cup	• right before pouring in molds
Cornmeal	1/4 cup	• right before pouring in molds
Ground almonds	1/4 cup	• right before pouring in molds
Mustard seeds	1/4 cup	• right before pouring in molds
Powdered oatmeal	1/4 cup	• right before pouring in molds
Seaweed	1/4 cup	• right before pouring in molds
Tapioca pearls	1 1/2 tsp	• right before pouring in molds

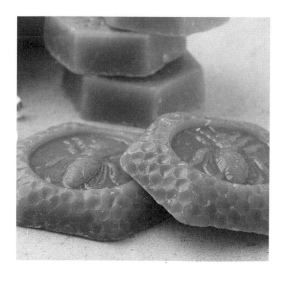

Waxes

Waxes are added primarily to stabilize and thicken the soap. It also helps contribute to the hardness of the final bar. Beeswax has the added bonus of giving your soap a faint honey smell.

ADDITIVE	HOW MUCH	WHEN TO ADD TO THE OIL/FAT BASE
Beeswax	1/4 cup	• melt with oil/fat base before adding lye/water mixture
Lanolin	3 tablespoons	• before adding lye/water mixture
Lecithin	2 1/2 tablespoons	• before adding lye/water mixture

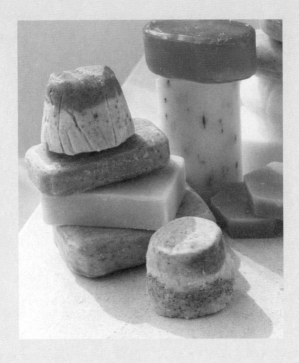

Making soap, just like cooking or any other activity that revolves around timing, attention and creativity, requires common sense, forethought and organization. With just a few simple guidelines, your soap making experience can be fun, safe and incredibly rewarding.

Safety Measures and Tips

The first thing you need to do after gathering your tools and supplies is to select a proper work area. Because of noxious lye fumes, it should be well ventilated (working outside is ideal), and away from household traffic, especially kids and pets. It's also a good idea to cover the work surface and surrounding floor with newspaper or cardboard to protect it from spills.

The next thing is to pick out your soap making outfit. If you're thinking sexy or sleek right now, I would advise changing activities. The first rule of thumb is that you want to cover your body as much as possible so as to avoid any contact between skin and lye. In other words, wearing shorts, a tank top and sandals is not recommended. A more practical attire would consist of a long-sleeved shirt, an old pair of sweats and closed-toe shoes.

Eye protection—either safety goggles or glasses—and gloves are an absolute must. The goggles will protect your eyes from lye fumes, and the gloves protect your hands from lye and heat. It's important to keep the gloves and goggles on at all times, even when handling the soap after it has hardened (when taking it out of molds, for example) as the lye will stay caustic until the aging process of the soap is complete (see page 49 to learn more about the aging process). A disposable facemask is strongly recommended for protecting against inhaling lye fumes. Just as with most activities, remove jewelry to avoid getting it dirty or damaging it. The fact that lye will corrode metal is another reason to abide by this rule.

When handling all soap-making ingredients, use common sense and follow safety precautions on the packaging. Specifically when handling lye, open the container only when you are ready to use it, and seal it immediately thereafter. Lye gets lumpy and loses some of its strength when in contact with air, and the goal is to minimize any potential spills and escaping fumes. It's also a good idea to keep a bottle of white vinegar or some lemon juice handy in case your skin comes into contact with lye, lye solution or liquid soap. The acidity of these ingredients will counteract the caustic effect of lye and re-establish the skin's natural pH balance. Apply the vinegar or lemon juice to the affected area (lye will first feel slimy on your skin, then it will start to itch and burn), rinse abundantly with water and pat dry. If lye or lye solution gets on the work area, wash immediately with soapy water, rinse well and wipe dry. When disposing of lye, follow safety precautions on the container or ask someone at your local hardware store. Remember to label the container in which you mix lye with water. That container should be used for soapmaking purposes only.

Write down all ingredients and measurements as you go along so that you can refer back to them if need be. Occasionally, you might be able to remedy a batch that has gone wrong, if you know where you went wrong and by how much.

Finally, no matter how good your soap might look or smell when you're making it, NEVER taste it, be extra careful about touching it with an unprotected hand and above all, be patient! The only good soap is a finely cured one.

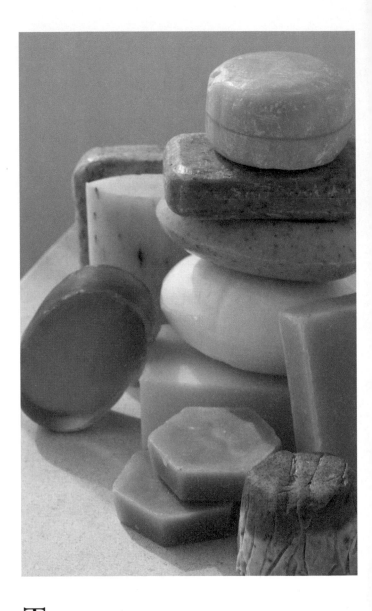

There are essentially three ways of making soap: cold-process, hand-milling and melting, which I call The Jell-O™ Method. Your schedule and patience will determine which technique will most likely suit your needs.

The Three Categories:

COLD-PROCESS is the method that is most similar to the way soap was traditionally made. Specifically, it revolves around a process known as saponification, which is a chemical reaction between an acid (animal fats or oils) and a base (lye, or sodium hydroxide, and water). When the acid and base meet, they eventually combine and form a thick, soupy mixture known as liquid soap. This mixture is then poured into molds and aged. The reason why this method is called cold-process reflects the fact that once the melted fats or oils and lye are combined, there is no need to add additional heat to the process. The mixtures "cook" on their own.

Cold-process is the most time-consuming process of the three— you are starting from scratch, and are taking on the responsibility of guiding the transformation from a collection of separate ingredients to a bar of soap. Purists might even opt to "render" their own tallow, which is a process by which animal fats are melted down and purified.

HAND-MILLED soaps are made from grated cold-process soaps, which are then melted and remolded. These soaps are smoother, last longer and are harder than the original cold-processed ones. Anyone on a tighter schedule or in need for more instant gratification—at the expense of quality and purity—can gather bits and pieces of leftover commercially manufactured soap, grate them, melt down and remold. It's actually a good way of getting rid of those slivers of soap that often end up making their way through the drain. But, then again, you don't get to enjoy the coddling process: watching lye, water and fats grow into an actual bar.

MELTING or THE JELL-O METHOD is the least time consuming and by far the simplest process of all. It involves melting down blocks of glycerin and pouring them into molds. Although the least traditional, this method is conducive to creativity and experimentation. More time can be spent on conjuring up ways of personalizing your glycerin bars: for example, you can drop various trinkets into the clear soap after pouring it into molds and before it sets—from little plastic toys (Barbie shoes or tiny farm animals) to fortune cookie fortunes, coffee beans, Bazooka Joe comics and decals, depending on your mood.

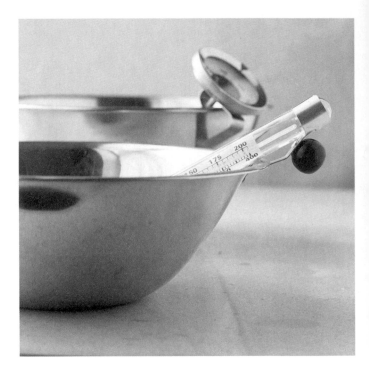

The key to making soap, especially the cold-process kind, is temperature control, which is why an accurate candy or cooking thermometer is essential. If your readings are not accurate, then you can forget about the quality of your soap.

In order to produce the desired chemical reaction between acid and base, the fats or oils and the lye solution need to be within a certain temperature range when blended together. The idea is to get them within 5°-10°F of each other. Both acid and base need to be between 95° and 100°F, with slight variations depending on the type of fat or oils used. Furthermore, it is important to remember that fats and oils do not heat at the same speed as the lye–water mixture. When you first combine sodium hydroxide (lye) with water, it takes a few minutes for it to completely dissolve but it starts to heat on its own right away. Very quickly—within a matter of minutes—the mixture will reach temperatures as high as 200° F and this is without applying direct heat! Fats and oils, on the other hand, can take longer, especially if the fats need to melt down before heating up. One suggested method is to let the lye mixture cool overnight and heat it up in a hot water bath (see below) at the last minute, just before pouring it into the fats or oils.

When monitoring the temperature of the various mixtures, there are a few things to keep in mind. If you're dealing with the fats or oils (and hence the application of heat to raise their temperature) make sure you give it a good stir so that the thermometer is reading the overall temperature. A thermometer that hangs on the side of the pot is far more accurate than one that sits on the bottom and hence records the heat of the flame. The temperature of the lye solution is in a sense easier to monitor as there is no external heat source to consider and the mixture homogeneously distributes the heat on its own.

With all that said, the only thing that is going to make this temperature control issue less daunting is practice and a bit of juggling, initially, but it's easy once you get a feel for the properties of your chosen ingredients.

Water baths—hot or cold—are very helpful in adjusting the temperature of mixtures. If your fats or oils get too hot for the lye solution, then a cold water bath will do the trick. And conversely for the lye solution: You can bring its temperature down by immersing it in a cold water bath.

To create a cold water bath, simply take a large bowl, pot or bucket and fill it halfway with cold water. Place the recipient of the oils/fats or lye solution and place it in the bath, making sure that none of the bath water gets into the mixture. Keep an eye on the thermometer until the temperature is within the proper range. When cooling down fats, remember that if water is too cold, fats may begin to congeal—or solidify—on the surface. To avoid a thin layer of solid fat, make sure you stir continuously until the desired temperature is reached.

A hot water bath raises or maintains the temperature of a liquid by immersing it in hot water. Again, immerse only enough of the container so that water doesn't get into the mixture. Monitor the temperature periodically.

You'll get the idea after a few batches and water baths will most likely become obsolete, but they're an incredibly useful tool at first.

The Saponification Process

As mentioned on page 13, saponification is a sophisticated term for describing the chemical reaction between lye and oil—the moment when your elements actually become soap. The best part about this stage is that you don't have to do anything except watch.

Chemically speaking, saponification is the result of the contact between an acid and a base, or a fat and an alkali. It is this contact which produces heat, soap and glycerin.

When combining the two mixtures, it's important to avoid splashes and spills, hence the importance of a container with a pouring spout which allows you to control the speed at which the lye solution is added to the oils. The lye mixture should be added in a steady stream while stirring continuously, and without splashing. The only thing to keep in mind is that saponification depends on a particular acid/base ratio, which varies with the type of acid used. In other words, not all fats or oils require the same amount of lye solution in order for saponification to occur. In fact, each fat or oil has a SAP value, or saponification value, which helps determine how much lye needs to be used to initiate saponification (see saponification chart on page 170). This is only something to consider when substituting one fat or oil in a recipe for another.

Tracing

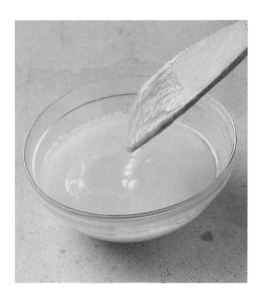

Tracing occurs just as that moment when the liquid soap has turned soupy and opaque, and you can "trace" a line or design on the surface of the soap when you pick up the spoon and let the liquid drizzle like icing. Signs of tracing are an indication that both mixtures have "saponified" and merged into one homogeneous substance. It signifies the formation of "liquid soap," which has the consistency of very watery but grainy mashed potatoes or thick soup. For anyone who enjoys cooking, saponification is that precise moment when the egg whites have peaked to perfection and become meringue or when the Béarnaise Sauce turns out just right.

Tracing can take anywhere from fifteen minutes to an hour and a half or even two, depending on the ingredients used. Soaps made out of animal fats tend to show signs of tracing much quicker than soaps made out of liquid vegetable oils. This is where and when you need to be particularly patient.

A vigorous stir will render the best saponification. The goal is to stir briskly enough so that the ingredients are well blended but not too briskly so as to create air bubbles in the liquid soap. However, if you're looking to make a soap that floats, now is the time to filter in all those air bubbles. Avoid using a hand mixer unless it is set on super slow speed.

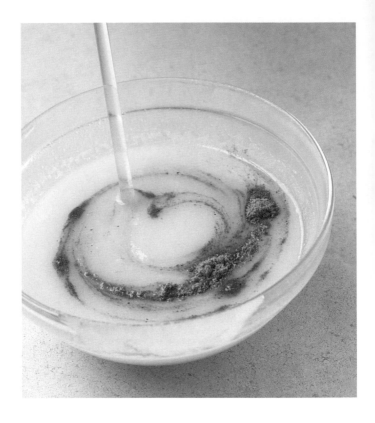

T his is where the really fun part comes in: personalizing your soap
by adding all sorts of ingredients to it. Almost anything is fair game:
from essential oils, to honey, herbs and dried fruit, depending on your
fancy. Just keep in mind that whatever you add should be chopped or
ground fine enough so as not to clog your bathtub's drain. Generally,
it's wise to avoid huge lumps or pieces of anything in your soap.
Chunky soap is not particularly fun to use.

At this stage, (post-tracing), the liquid soap should still be warm.
Whatever you add to the liquid soap should be at a reasonably warm
temperature so that the liquid doesn't go into shock when the bits and
pieces of ingredients are added to it. It's not essential to actually heat
up these ingredients; just remember to take them out of the refrigerator so that they at least reach room temperature before blending
them into the liquid soap.

Then the question "what to add?" arises. The following are just a
few suggestions. Let your imagination go wild.

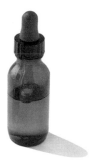

HEALING CHARACTERISTICS: Essential oils are the extract or pure "essence" of plants, bark, flowers, leaves, grasses, or stems and carry specific and distinct healing properties. Highly volatile in nature, these oils can be added directly to the liquid soap, either alone or in combination form. Remember that a little goes a very long way as these oils are highly concentrated. Generally one to three tablespoons of essential oil per batch of soap is sufficient. (See essential oil chart on pages 165–67.)

SCENT: Fragrance oils are synthetic blends with an alcohol base. These can be a bit tricky to work with as they tend to accelerate the tracing process so the liquid soap thickens quickly. Make sure you are ready to pour the soap into the molds shortly after having added the fragrance oils. Certain fragrance oils have even been known to interfere with the saponification process. It's preferable to do a "test" batch before adding any fragrance oil to the entire pot.

COLOR: A soap's color can be achieved either naturally or chemically. There are various chemical dyes on the market available from soap supply companies. Another way of coloring soap is by using crayons. Crayons are made out of wax and can be melted before adding them to the liquid soap. One crayon is sufficient to color one batch of soap.

Personally, I prefer to stick to the more traditional methods of coloring soap which give the bars a more subtle hue and a "natural" appeal. Approximately one tablespoon of the finely ground ingredient will be enough to color one batch of soap. Make sure all ingredients are either very finely ground or strained. Also keep in mind that the color will lighten as the soap sets. See the color examples on the following pages for ideas.

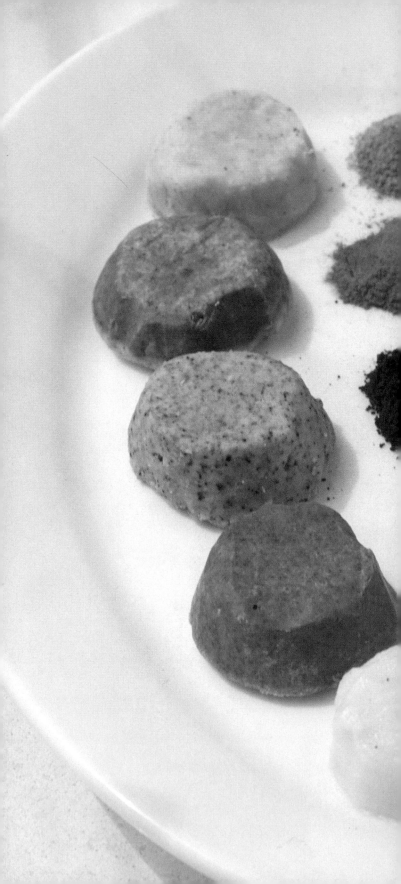

- **Curry Powder**

- **Cinnamon**

- **Coffee Grounds**

- **Paprika**

- **Crayon**

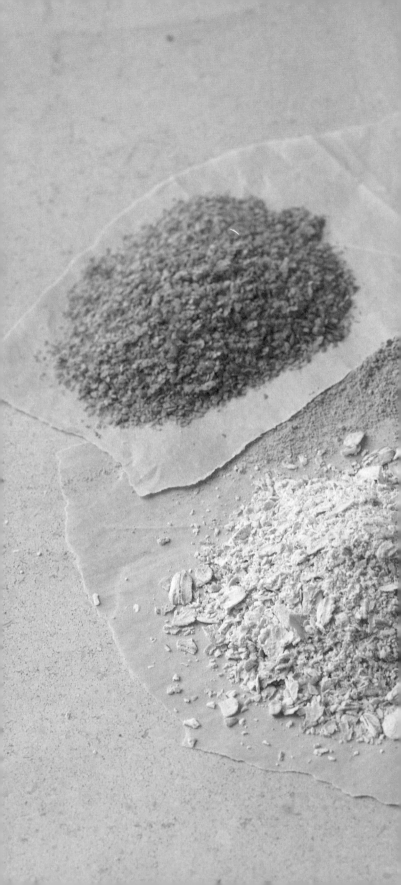

Custom Blends

DESIRED COLOR OR HUE	INGREDIENT
green	• liquid green chlorophyll • strained spinach baby food
orange	• strained carrot baby food
peach	paprika
yellow gold	curry powder turmeric
burnt orange	• ground henna
brown	• coca powder • ground dark chocolate • finely ground coffee
beige	cinnamon powder nutmeg powder
pinkish-orange	• cayenne pepper
reddish-pink	strained mashed cooked beets concentrated beet juice

TEXTURE: When adding any ingredients to your liquid soap, it's important to remember that you don't want your soap to be clogging your drains and you certainly don't want to feel like you're washing with popcorn or trail mix. Therefore, finely grind or thoroughly chop whatever you will be adding.

TRY ADDING:
• Finely chopped or grated fresh or dried fruits, citrus peels, fresh or dried flowers and petals, nuts and vegetables to add character, density, and color herbs and spices for color and texture

Skin Exfoliants:
• Clay, ground wheat germ, ground oatmeal, cornstarch, dried or fresh seaweed, tapioca pearls

Skin Softeners:
• Milk (cow or goat's milk), cream, honey, vitamin E or lanolin

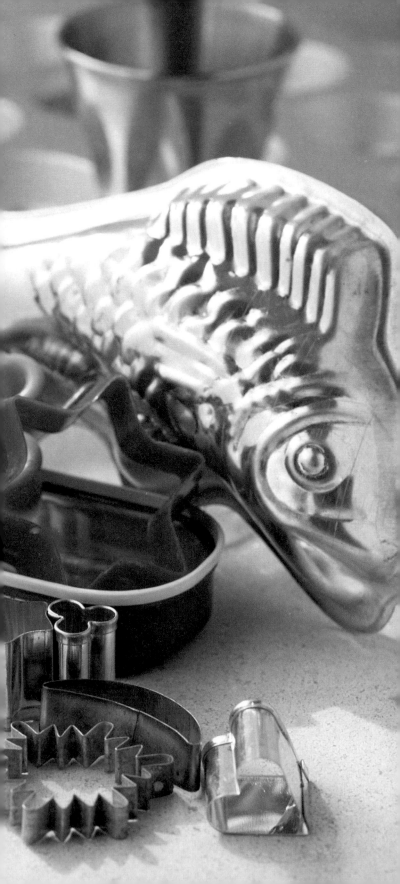

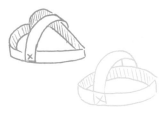

Soap molds fall into two categories: molds, and anything else that might work as a mold but was probably never intended to be one.

MOLDS: If you're looking to make a more sophisticated and fancy bar, traditional molds will best suit your needs. Although you can purchase molds specifically intended for soap making in supply stores, your best bet is the candy, cookie or cake mold isle at the nearest K-Mart™, or local craft-supply store. Whatever shape you select, make sure you pick one that won't make the soap too small or too narrow because you don't want it to slide down the drain.

The rule of thumb—and this applies to non-traditional molds as well—is that you are looking for molds that are not made out of aluminum, zinc, copper, Teflon™ or iron, as these will corrode when in contact with lye. Corrosion does not necessarily affect the quality of the soap but certainly does the effectiveness of the mold the next time you use it. Ceramic, stainless steel, plastic, rubber, ovenproof stoneware, china or glass molds are ideal for making soaps. Whether using small soufflé dishes or chocolate molds, the material must be able to withstand the heat of liquid soap. Basically, if the mold can withstand very hot mashed potatoes, it will work.

Prepare your soap molds before you start anything else. You don't want to be caught with a vat of warm liquid soap that's ready to be poured and no mold to pour it into.

In order to insure that your soap won't stick to the mold, you must grease it first, with non-stick vegetable spray or Crisco™. Another option is to line the mold with plastic wrap or wax paper, in lieu of spray or shortening. You also want to make sure that your molds are at least at room temperature when you pour liquid soap into them so as to avoid any temperature shock if the molds are too cold.

After you have poured the liquid soap into the mold, put a sheet of plastic wrap over it. This minimizes the contact of the soap with air, thus diminishing "soda ash" (see Troubleshooting, page 100).

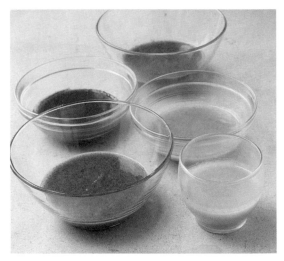

ANYTHING ELSE THAT MIGHT WORK
AS A MOLD BUT WAS PROBABLY NEVER
INTENDED TO BE ONE:

Be creative! Many soapmakers in fact prefer these "less-traditional" molds. Many of them are disposable and flexible, which makes any unmolding difficulties moot. If the soap won't come out, then just peel or cut the mold right off. But the important thing to remember when selecting molds is that, similar to traditional molds, these need to withstand the heat of the liquid soap.

Whether your mold is plastic, rubber, or wood, it needs to be lined in one way or another. Plastics, rubber, glass, ceramic or clay should be sprayed with a non-stick vegetable spray or greased with Crisco™ as with the traditional soap molds.

If your mold is cardboard or wood, it should also be lined. You can use plastic wrap by spreading it carefully along the bottom of the mold and folding it over the side, ensuring that there are no air bubbles trapped between the plastic and the mold. Wax paper is also effective as a liner. You'll need tape to secure the edges of the paper to the molds. Lining in this fashion also makes the unmolding process a lot easier. Simply pull up the sides of the plastic film or wax paper and voilá! The soap is out.

Here are a few suggestions for non-traditional molds:

- *plastic ice cube trays*
- *shoe boxes*
- *wood boxes*
- *shirt boxes*
- *heavy cardboard boxes*
- *plastic drawer organizers*
- *anything Tupperware*
- *milk cartons*
- *tuna or sardine cans (the ones that are lined with a plastic film)*
- *Jell-O Jiggler molds*
- *plastic sand toys or sand castle molds*
- *plastic Easter eggs (the kind used for Easter egg hunts that come apart)*
- *clay flower pots*
- *storage containers*
- *PVC pipe (available in hardware stores) for making soaps that look like hockey pucks*

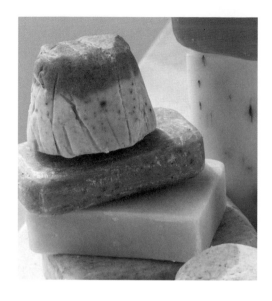

After you have poured the liquid soap into the molds, it's essential to cover the surface with plastic wrap (or a plastic garbage bag) so as to minimize the chemical reaction between air and lye in the soap. The plastic wrap must be taut on the soap's surface. If you are using a plastic storage container with a lid, put the lid on after you have stretched the plastic wrap over the soap. Instead of plastic wrap, you can also use a piece of wood or heavy cardboard that completely covers the top of the mold.

Cover the molds with blankets or towels. This is the initial stage of the curing and insulation period. The purpose of this stage is to cool the soap at a steady rate and to allow the saponification process to continue. If the soap cools too quickly, it will become fragile and fray easily (see Troubleshooting page 100). During the cooling period— which can take from 16 to 24 hours depending on the ingredients used—all you have to do is wait. If you're overcome with desire to handle the soap at this point (which is not advised), make sure you have your rubber gloves on as the saponification process is still in effect and the lye remains caustic.

After this initial cooling process, uncover the molds and let them sit in a dark place that is free from drafts and cold for another three to six days. Since not all soaps harden at the same pace (soaps made with beeswax, for example, tend to harden quickly), it's a good

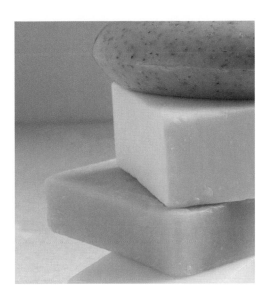

idea to peek at your soap every once in a while to test how it's doing. Remember to have your rubber gloves on when you poke at it, as the saponification process is not yet complete.

Once the soap is firm enough that you can cut it and it will retain its shape, remove it from the mold. Do not wait until it is completely hard, though, or you will not be able to cut it at all. If you find that the surface of the soap is very liquid and oily, then you might have encountered a separation problem. (See Trouble-shooting, page 99).

If you have used individual molds, the soap should come out—like ice from a tray or muffins from a pan—with a little coaxing. As long as your soap is hard enough, it should be able to withstand a little wiggling. Sometimes, even greased molds are hard to unmold, especially with porous materials such as china or clay. In that case, place the mold in the freezer for about half an hour. The soap will "sweat" and should come right out.

If you used a shirt, shoe, cardboard box or any other type of mold that is larger than you want your soap to be in the end, you'll want to cut the slab of soap into individual bars. If you don't care about pre-serving the mold, you can cut the soap into bars right through the mold, then discard the mold and separate the pieces. Or, you can remove the entire block of soap from the mold and then cut it.

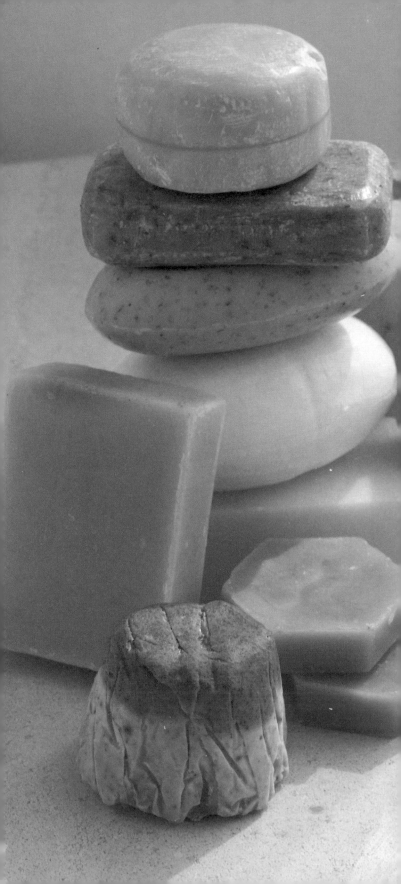

SITTING, COOLING AND AGING

T he key is to get to the soap when it starts having the consistency of Swiss cheese. If you wait too long, then the soap will be too hard to cut. If you don't wait long enough, then your soap will be too soft to slice into. It takes some probing, common sense and practice to get it just right.

Once the soap is hard enough to slice, take a ruler or template and slice into the block with a very sharp knife. Trim off any irregular bumps or rough edges. Your soap will take its final form during the next aging period, so do any trimming or smoothing now.

Very often, as soap is curing, a fine layer of white, chalky soda ash will accumulate on the surface. Don't be alarmed, it's just a byproduct of the contact with air—just wipe it off with a damp rag (gloves on!), run it under cold water and then pat it dry or scrape it off with a paring knife.(If you find that there is an abundance of soda ash, refer to Troubleshooting, page 100, for tips on how to avoid it in the next batch.) Once cut and trimmed, place the individual bars on a piece of wax paper, brown paper bag, or drying rack. (Remember: You still need to have your gloves on!)

Again, store your soap in a dark, dry place, free of drafts and temperature changes. This aging process is the second stage of curing (the first one being when the soap is covered with blanket or towels), which furthers the process by which the pH in the soap stabilizes. This cure, which lasts three to four weeks, is what makes the soap mild and hard. About half way into the aging process, turn the soaps over so that both sides are equally exposed to air.

*Congratulations! You have just completed
your first batch of soap!*

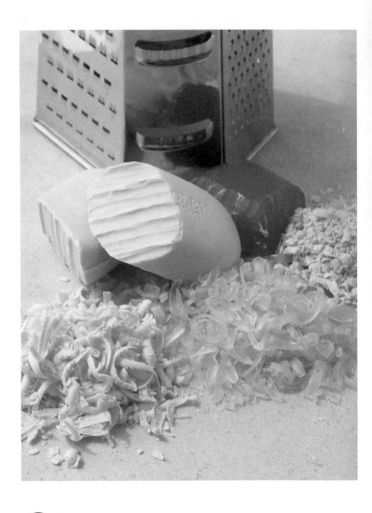

Once you've made cold-process soap, making hand-milled soap is truly a piece of cake. Hand milling involves three easy steps: grating soap, melting it and remolding it. That's it!

The purpose of hand-milling soap is to create a bar that is longer lasting, harder and smoother than its cold-processed counter part, and it's an opportunity to enjoy the creative side of soapmaking on a shorter schedule than cold-process.

When grating soap, you are dealing with a product that has already completed its saponification process and aging stage. Therefore, one of the many advantages of making hand-milled soap is that you can add whatever ingredients you want to the grated soap to personalize it (essential oils, milk, honey, oatmeal, dyes, teas, spices, fruit, etc.), without worrying about how it might affect the lye or the saponification process. Words such as tracing, separating, curdling or curing are definitely not a part of the hand-miller's vocabulary.

Another tremendous advantage of making hand-milled soap is that it enables you to revamp a batch of cold-process soap. If, for some reason, your cold-process soap came out not quite as you expected, this is the perfect opportunity to grate it, melt it, breathe some new life into it and remold it.

Furthermore, hand-milling is the ideal way by which to get rid of those little pieces of left-over soap that are too small to use but too large to slip down the drain. Simply save those little soap odds and ends in a container, and once you have a fair about a pound, start grating!

The recipe for making hand-milled soap is extremely easy and requires very little equipment, save a cheese grater (or a food processor) and a double boiler. You'll also need approximately 12 ounces of liquid (milk, tea or water) for every pound of grated soap. You should use a basic soap (see Basic Vegetable Soap, page 64).

First, prepare your molds as you would for cold-process making soap, by spraying them with a non-stick vegetable spray or by greasing them with vegetable shortening. In a double boiler, heat whatever liquid you choose (milk, buttermilk, water and honey mixture, herbal tea, plain water, dyed water) to 170° F to 180° F. Add the grated soap, stirring slowly but constantly. Reduce heat so that the liquid and grated soap come to a gentle simmer, stirring regularly—but not constantly—until all of the grated soap is liquefied. Then add your ingredients and additives (oatmeal, spices, herbs, flowers, cornmeal, clay, coffee, seaweed, lanolin, cocoa butter, essential oils, fragrance oils, etc.) and stir to blend. Immediately ladle or pour mixture into molds and cover with plastic wrap. After 24 hours, remove plastic wrap and set molds in a draft-free dry place for three to four weeks.

Keep in mind that whatever ingredients are added to the liquefied grated soap–water mixture will affect the final consistency and texture of the soap. The amount of ingredients you use is a matter of personal preference. Generally, use approximately 1/2 ounce of essential or fragrance oil to every pound of grated soap. For dry ingredients, approximately 1/2 cup to every pound of grated soap should do.

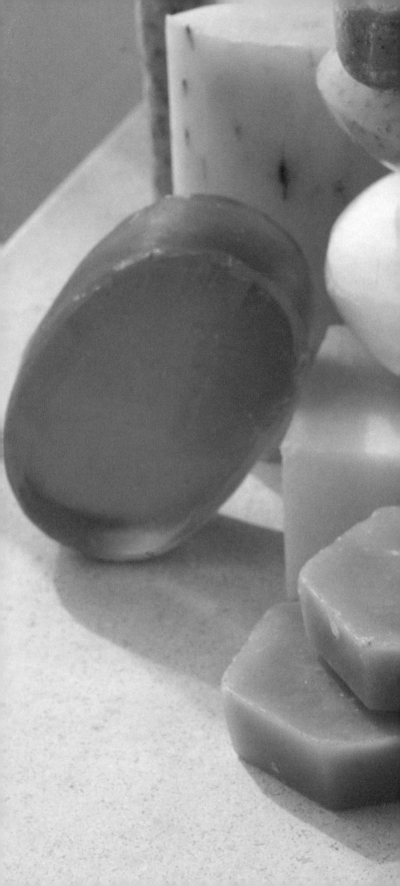

The Jell-O™ Method

The reason why I refer to this as "the Jell-O™ Method" is because if you've ever made Jell-O™, you'll be a pro at this process. Essentially, the melting method is two-step process: melting down a block of store-bought glycerin and pouring into molds.

There are many advantages to making soaps using this method. First of all, because you are dealing with glycerin—and not lye or a lye mixture—there are none of the safety concerns that you have when making cold-processed soap. It also means that you can pretty much use whatever mold you want (provided the mold is heat-resistant) since there is no possibility of corrosion. Second, this process takes very little time and the gratification is practically instantaneous. There is no saponification, tracing, curing, or aging to worry about. Simply melt, pour, wait for it to harden and unmold. Third, because glycerin is translucent, you can virtually go wild with ways to personalize your soap.

Prepare your molds in the same way as you would for making cold-process soap by spraying them with a non-stick vegetable spray or coating them with vegetable shortening. After having broken up your slab of glycerin into pieces, place them in a double boiler and melt until fully liquefied. Remove from heat. Add personalizing ingredients: flower petals, dyes, essential and fragrance oils (approximately 1/2 ounce per pound of glycerin), herbs, spices, coconut flakes, grated lemon peel, sparkles, etc. Ladle or pour into molds and let sit in a draft-free dry place for approximately twenty-four hours or until soap is completely hard. Remove from molds.

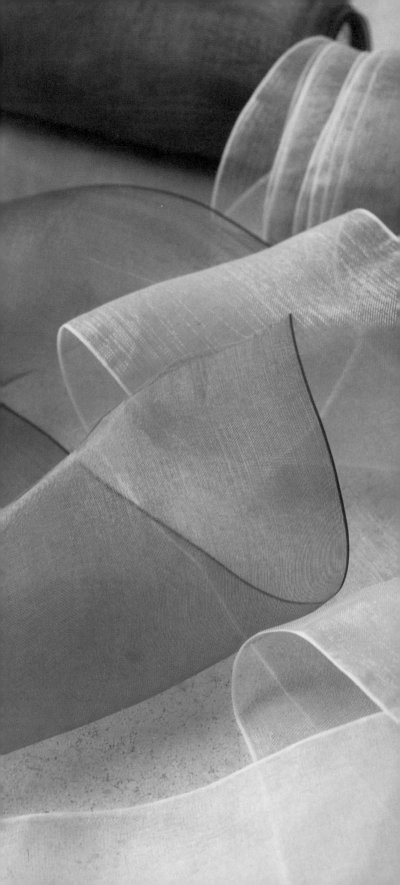

Decorating soap is just as much fun as making it. This is really an effective way of personalizing your soaps and exploring your own ideas

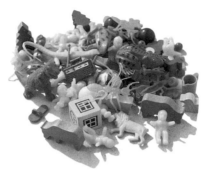

Hidden Treasures

Decoration can come into play at various stages of the soap making process. When you're pouring soap into molds, you can embed charms, trinkets, small toys, little messages or fortune cookie fortunes in your soap. Fill up the mold halfway, place whatever treasure you want in your soap in the middle and gently pour the rest of the liquid in to fill the mold. You may also ease a toy or trinket into a full mold with a glass rod, knife or chopstick—but be sure that you've left a little space at the top so the mold doesn't overflow. This technique is especially useful when you're making soap with the Jell-O™ Method, and the end result will be a clear, glycerin soap, so you can see what's inside. The possibilities are endless, but here are a few ideas to get you started:

- *fortune cookie fortunes*
- *plastic Barbie™ accessories*
- *miniature plastic animals or toys*
- *coffee beans*
- *dried whole flowers*
- *four-leaf clovers*
- *cinnamon drops*
- *pieces of vanilla bean*
- *dried fruit and nuts*
- *charms*
- *beads*

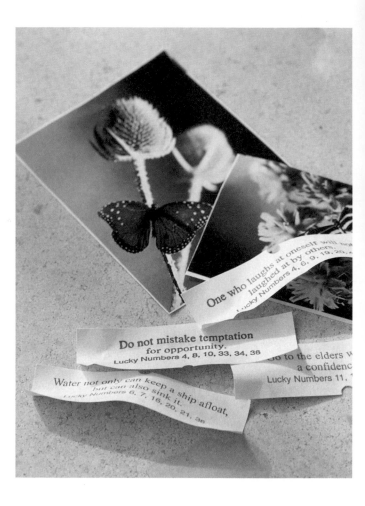

If, on the other hand, you want to decorate the surface of the soap by applying something to it or imprinting something on it, then you should do so during the final stage of the aging process, but just before the soap has completely hardened. As you become more comfortable with each soapmaking stage, you'll quickly learn to recognize when the time is right. Initially, you might have to periodically test the soap to see if it's ready for your personal signature. Test the side of the soap first to see if the surface is hard enough to sustain an imprint.

There are several ways to make imprints on soap. You can use cookie stamps, for example, or wax sealing stamps (the kind used to seal envelopes) which add an antique look to the finished soap. Make sure you have greased the stamp or sprayed with non-stick vegetable spray before using it so it will make a clean impression and not stick.

You can also press something into the surface of the soap at this particular time (like an almond, vanilla bean, or small piece of chocolate) for a unique effect.

Applying decals is another fun way of giving character to your soap. The decal-applying process is done after the final curing period is complete. You can essentially "paste" any image, picture or word(s) on the surface of your soap with the help of a little paraffin wax and mineral oil. Simply melt a small amount of paraffin wax (you can even use a crayon) in a saucepan over low heat. Place the "decal" (cut out from magazines, catalogs, wrapping paper, cards, etc,) on the soap's surface and with a paintbrush fix it to the soap with the melted paraffin wax. Once the wax has completely hardened, gently rub the decal with a bit of mineral oil to remove a layer of the wax to bring the decal to the surface. As you use the soap, the decal will wash away, but it makes for a great first impression as a gift.

Soap Balls

Making soap balls is just like making snow balls. The key is to be handling the soap (with gloves on!) after the initial curing or cooling down period, when the soap is till warm. Simply scoop out a handful of soap and roll it around in the palm of your hands until it forms a ball. At this point, you can roll it into shaved white soap (for a real snowball effect) or into finely ground oatmeal, lavender flowers, crushed dried rose petals or herbs, for example.

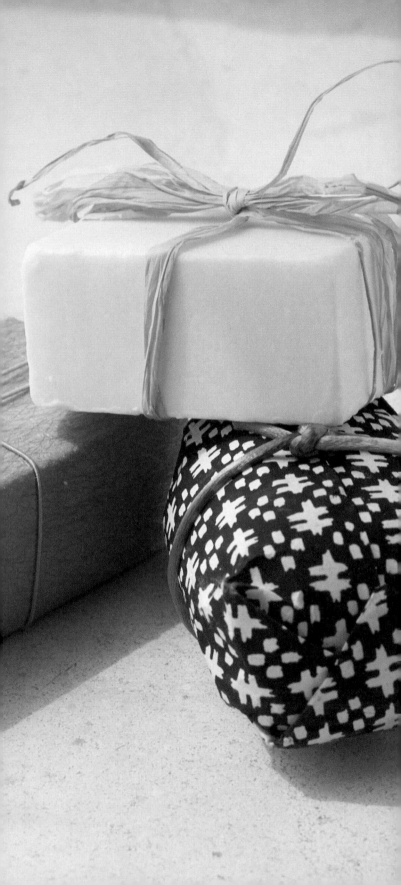

There is no rule of thumb for packaging soap except that you should use breathable materials (tissue paper, brown paper, fabric, or wood, for example). If your soap is particularly fragrant, you should wrap it as quickly as possible after the curing process is complete so as to retain its scent. Anything beyond that is just a matter of aesthetics and taste. (In fact, you don't have to wrap your soap to store it, provided you keep it in a cool, dry and dark place.)

The packaging material you select will depend on what look you want to give your soap. For a wholesome and natural look, twine, dried banana leaves, raffia or handcrafted writing paper work well. Ribbons, printed fabrics and silk, on the other hand, add a sophisticated finish to the final product. Tissue paper, lace, or tulle can be more coquettish and delicate. You'll quickly discover that packaging possibilities are endless and you'll be amazed by what you come up with!

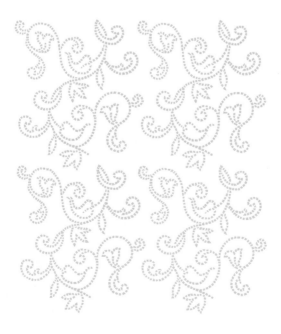

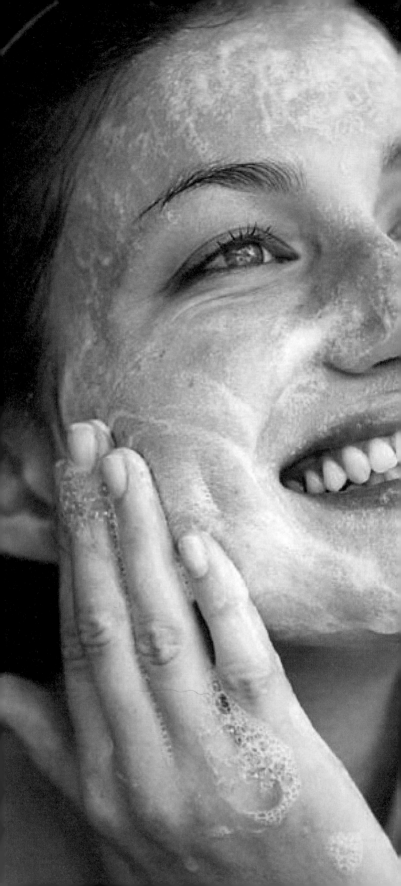

Soap Recipes

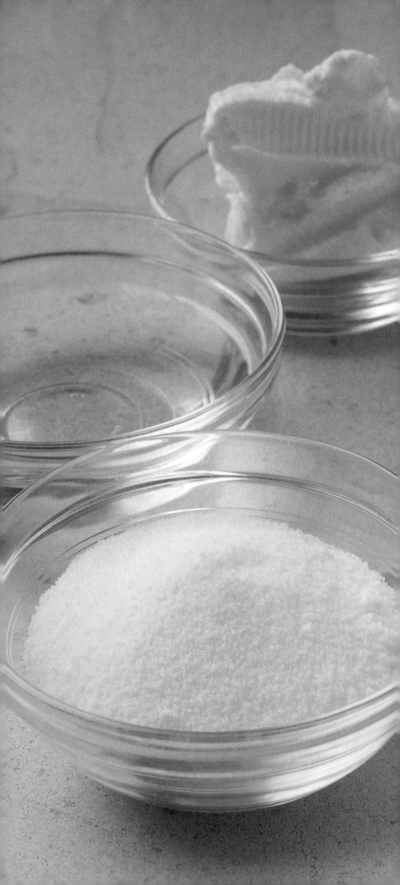

BASIC SOAPS

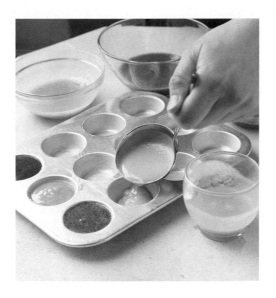

Most custom recipes can be made with either vegetable oils or animal fat. Because vegetable oils are often easier to work with and more predictable, the custom blends offered here use a vegetable oil soap as a base. I have provided a basic animal fat recipe as well, which can be used interchangeably with the vegetable base—choose whichever method you prefer.

All measurements are given in weights, not volumes

These recipes yield approximately ten to twelve bars of hand soap, or about 3 pounds of soap

Basic Vegetable Soap

This white or off-white vegetable soap makes an ideal base for making any personalized soap. You can add fragrances, color, texturing ingredients or virtually any other additives without worrying about affecting the soaps basic cleansing and moisturizing properties.

Olive oil–rich in minerals, proteins and vitamins–yields a healing, emollient soap that lathers in small, rich bubbles. The oil, notorious for helping the soap harden and dry quickly during the soap making process, also serves as an excellent base for essential or fragrance oils. Coconut oil, an odorless oil that hardens at room temperature, is a quick-lathering cleanser that is rapidly absorbed by the skin. Vegetable shortening gives the soap body and works well in the saponification process. Remember, you can further personalize your soap by substituting one (or all) of these oils for others, provided you check the SAP chart (see Saponification Chart, page 170) to adjust the amount of lye needed in the recipe.

Ingredients:

12 OUNCES COCONUT OIL

12 OUNCES OLIVE OIL

20 OUNCES VEGETABLE SHORTENING

16 OUNCES WATER, PREFERABLY DISTILLED
AND AT ROOM TEMPERATURE

6 OUNCES LYE

- Grease soap molds and set aside. Place coconut oil, olive oil and vegetable shortening in a large lye resistant and heat resistant pot. Heat the fats and stir regularly to dissipate heat. When the oils have reached a temperature within the 97°F to 100°F range, remove pot from heat.
- Place water in a lye resistant pitcher, preferably one with a pourable spout.
- With rubber gloves and safety goggles on, measure lye and slowly pour into water.
- Stir constantly but slowly with a stainless steel or wooden spoon until all lye is fully dissolved.
- When lye/water mixture is within the 97°F to 100°F range

(same as the temperature of the oils), start pouring lye/water mixture into oils in a thin and steady stream, while stirring occasionally. (To lower or raise temperature of oils or lye/water mixture, see Water Baths, page 33).

- Keep stirring constantly and slowly, but not over zealously. You don't want to be creating air bubbles in the mixture— unless you want your soap to float.

- After about 10 to 15 minutes, the mixture should start tracing, which means that it has gone from clear to opaque, that it has thickened and that when you now pick up the spoon in the pot, the liquid soap drizzles off of it and leaves a trace on the surface. If after 45 minutes to an hour, your soap mixture still hasn't started tracing yet, then you might have to recheck your measurements (see Troubleshooting, page 98).

- At this point, the soap mixture is ready to be poured or ladled into the molds. Do so, seal the mold with plastic wrap (or with the cover to the mold), put some blankets or towels on it and place it in a draft-free place. Let it sit for 48 hours.

- After 48 hours, remove the mold's lid and plastic wrap and assess your soap: with rubber gloves on (remember: the lye is still highly caustic so don't touch your soap with bare hands!) gently touch the surface of the soap. If the soap is still very soft, let it sit overnight and the next day unwrapped. If the soap is firm to the touch (yet still leaves an imprint) take the soap out of the mold cut into pieces (if necessary), trim off any excess and place it on a drying rack, clean butcher block or piece of plastic wrap.

- If you have used individual soap molds, then you simply need to wait another three weeks for your soap to have completed its aging process. If you have used a large mold and are planning on slicing it up into small bars, then start checking the soap after about one week or so.

- Once the soap is sliced, place the individual bars onto a drying rack, butcher block, a piece of plastic wrap or wax paper, and let the soap air dry for another 2½ weeks or until the surface of the soap is very hard to the touch. Scrape off whatever ash might be on the bar's surface with a sharp knife, and your soap is ready to use!

Basic Animal Fat Soap

Animal fat yields a mild bar that is much harder and lasts longer than its vegetable counterpart. Animal fat, tallow in particular, traces readily and dries easily. It's a multi-purpose soap that blends well with additives and has a creamy, mild lather. It's a good straightforward soap for beginners to make. To avoid graininess or discoloration in the soap, make sure the tallow you use is very clean.

Ingredients:

- 2 1/2 POUNDS OF BEEF TALLOW
- 16 OUNCES OF WATER, PREFERABLY DISTILLED AND AT ROOM TEMPERATURE
- 5 1/2 OUNCES OF LYE

DIRECTIONS:

- Grease soap molds and set aside.

- Place tallow in a large lye resistant pot and heat fat, stirring occasionally, until it reaches 120°F to 125°F.

- Place water in a lye resistant pitcher, preferably one with a pourable spout.

- With rubber gloves and safety goggles on, measure lye and slowly pour into water.

- Stir constantly but slowly with a stainless steel or wooden spoon until all lye is fully dissolved.

- When lye–water mixture is within the same temperature range as the tallow (between 120°F and 125°F), start pouring lye–water mixture into oils in a thin and steady stream, stirring occasionally. Refer to Basic Vegetable Soap recipe on page 64 for directions on saponification, tracing, cooling and aging.

Custom
Soaps

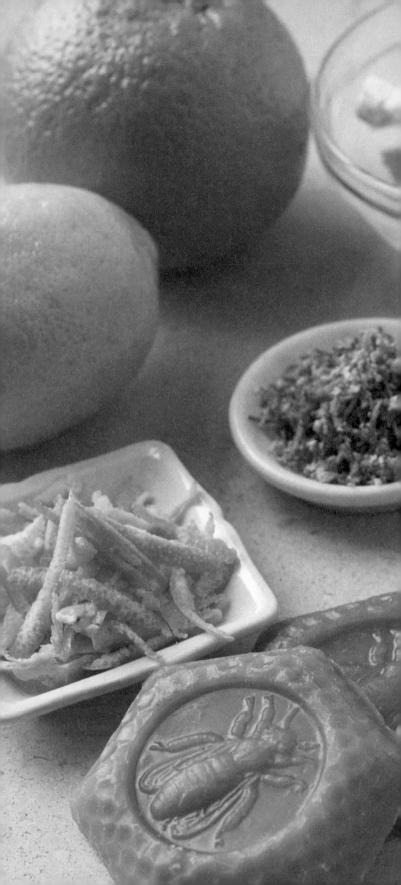

Summer Citrus Soap

This soap has a wonderfully uplifting and fresh smell to it, which makes it ideal for summer mornings. It has a firm consistency, rich lather and a golden hue from the beeswax.

Ingredients:

- INGREDIENTS FOR BASIC VEGETABLE SOAP
- 2 OUNCES BEESWAX
- 15 DROPS ORANGE ESSENTIAL OIL
- 10 DROPS LIME ESSENTIAL OIL
  OR LEMON ESSENTIAL OIL
- 1/4 CUP FINELY GRATED LIME PEEL
- 1/2 CUP FINELY GRATED LEMON
  OR ORANGE PEEL

- *Follow instructions for Basic Vegetable Soap, adding beeswax to oils and vegetable shortening so that they heat up and melt together before blending them with the water–lye solution.*
- *Just after the soap mixture has started tracing, quickly add essential oils and grated citrus peel.*
- *Stir until all ingredients are well blended.*
- *Pour mixture into greased molds and cover with a blanket or towel.*
- *Follow aging and drying instructions (see Sitting, Cooling and Aging).*

DON'T FORGET TO LABEL YOUR SOAP AFTER POURING IT INTO MOLDS. INCLUDE THE DATE OF MANUFACTURE, THE DATE THAT AGING PROCESS WAS COMPLETE AND THE INGREDIENTS THAT YOU USED.

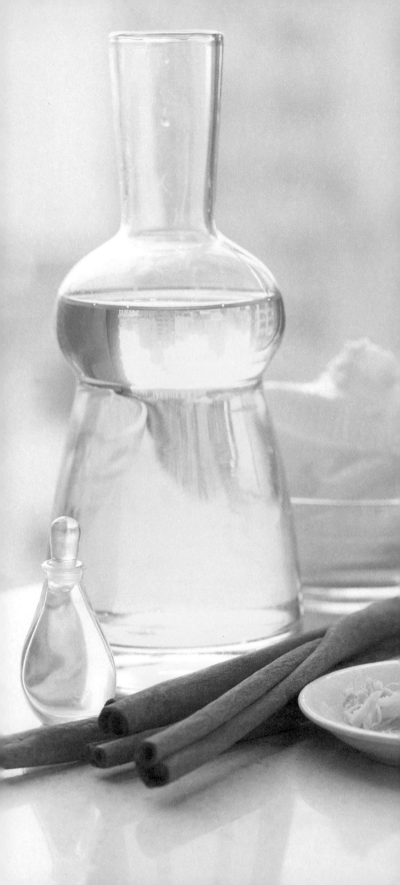

Cinnamon Ginger Soap

This soap is particularly invigorating and has a nice soft speckled brown note to it because of the cinnamon. The ginger has a warming effect on the skin and should not be used on sensitive or irritated skin.

Ingredients:

- INGREDIENTS FOR BASIC VEGETABLE SOAP
- 1 TEASPOON GROUND CINNAMON
- 2 TABLESPOONS FINELY GRATED GINGER
- 1/2 OUNCE GINGER ESSENTIAL OIL

- *Follow instructions for Basic Vegetable Soap.*
- *Just after the soap mixture has started to trace, add cinnamon, ginger and ginger essential oil.*
- *Stir until well blended and pour into greased molds. Follow aging and drying instructions (see Sitting, Cooling and Aging).*

SCENTED SOAPS SHOULD BE WRAPPED
TO AVOID DISSIPATION AND EVAPORATION
OF THE ESSENTIAL OILS.

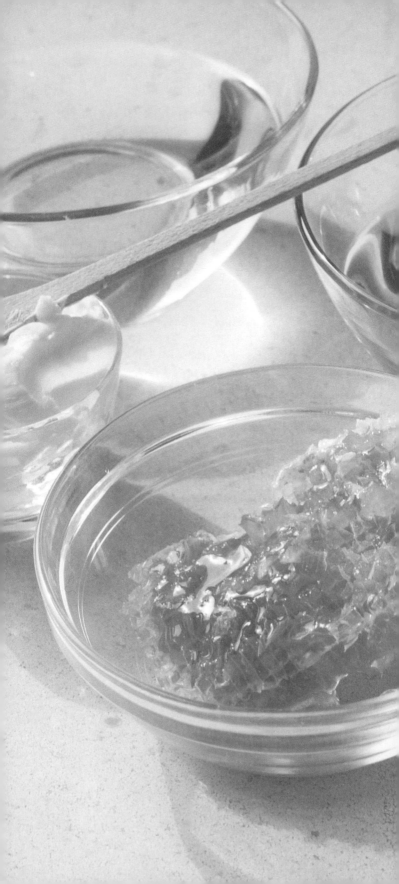

Soothing Honey Vanilla Soap

In addition to being soothing and moisturizing to the skin, this bar has a delicious honey-vanilla aroma that will make you want to eat it for breakfast. The beeswax will lend a warm golden tone to the soap.

Ingredients:

INGREDIENTS FOR BASIC VEGETABLE SOAP
2 OUNCES SWEET ALMOND OIL
6 OUNCES BEESWAX
1 OUNCE HONEY (SLIGHTLY WARMED)
2 OUNCES VANILLA ESSENTIAL OIL

- *Follow instructions for Basic Vegetable Soap, adding beeswax to the fats when you are heating them up.*

- *As soon as soap mixture begins to trace, add sweet almond oil, vanilla essential oil and the honey.*

- *Blend thoroughly and pour into molds.*

- *Follow aging and drying instructions (see Sitting, Cooling and Aging).*

RECIPES CAN BE DOUBLED OR TRIPLED, PROVIDED
YOU ACCURATELY ADJUST MEASUREMENTS.

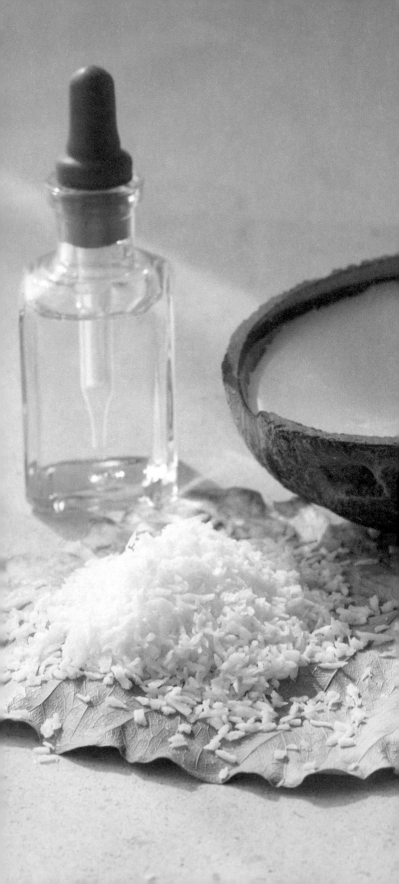

Smooth Coconut Rosewood Soap

Rosewood essential oil is noted for its calming and stress-reducing properties. It also has a nice spicy scent to it that blends perfectly with the subtle sweetness of coconut. This soap is ideal for all skin types and all times of day.

Ingredients:

INGREDIENTS FOR BASIC VEGETABLE SOAP

2 TABLESPOONS VERY FINELY GRATED COCONUT

3 OUNCES ROSEWOOD ESSENTIAL OIL

- *Follow instructions for Basic Vegetable Soap.*

- *As soon as soap mixture begins to trace, blend in essential oil and grated coconut.*

- *Pour into molds.*

- *Follow aging and drying instructions (see Sitting, Cooling and Aging).*

DO NOT INSULATE MORE THAN TWO TRAYS OF SOAP UNDER THE SAME BLANKET OR WRAP AT THE SAME TIME; THE UNEVEN DISTRIBUTION OF HEAT TO THE CENTER BARS MIGHT CAUSE THEM TO CURDLE.

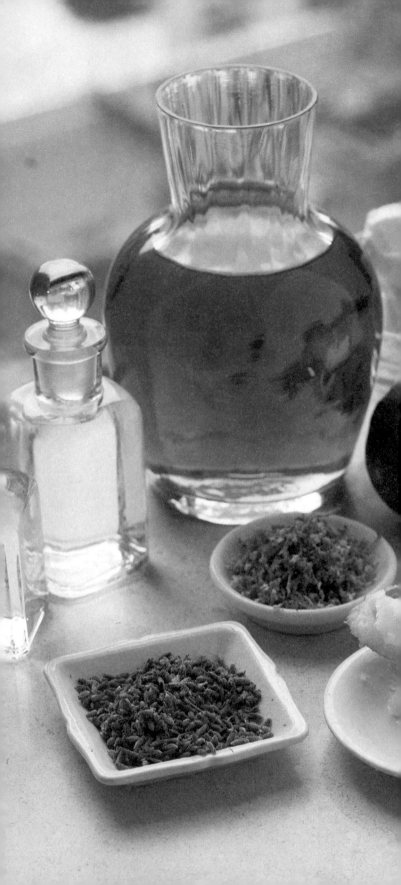

Cleansing Lavender Key Lime Soap

Called the universal oil because of its universal benefits, lavender oil will soothe and heal irritated skin. Its floral and clean smell is balancing and calming. Combined with the freshness of key lime, this bar is ideal for morning showers and baths. The grated peel and lavender flowers give the bar a beautiful color.

Ingredients:

INGREDIENTS FOR BASIC VEGETABLE SOAP

1 OUNCE LAVENDER ESSENTIAL OIL

1 OUNCE LIME ESSENTIAL OIL

2 TABLESPOONS FINELY GRATED KEY LIME
OR LIME PEEL

2 TABLESPOONS FINELY GRATED
DRIED LAVENDER

1 ½ OUNCES LIQUID CHLOROPHYLL
(FOR COLOR)

- Follow instructions for Basic Vegetable Soap.

- As soon as soap mixture begins to trace, add liquid chlorophyll and give it a good stir. Then blend in essential oils, grated lime peel and dried lavender.

- Mix thoroughly and pour into molds. Follow aging and drying instructions (see Sitting, Cooling and Aging).

ALWAYS WRITE DOWN YOUR MEASUREMENTS
AND INGREDIENTS. YOU MIGHT NEED TO REFER TO
THEM AT SOME LATER POINT.

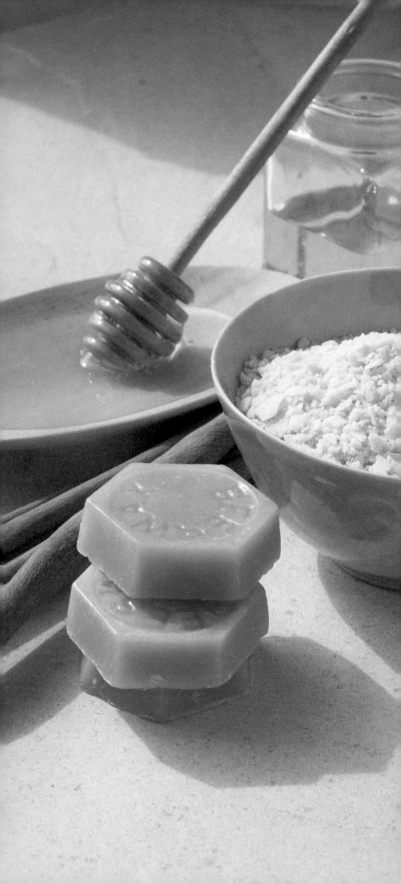

Moisturizing Honey Almond Soap with Nutmeg

T his soap has a dual function: mild exfolliant and skin moisturizer. Finely ground almonds serve as a mild abrasive gently removing dead surface cells, while honey moisturizes the skin and adds richness to the final bar. Sweet almond oil ensures a stable lather, and cinnamon provides a touch of color. Nutmeg, as an essential oil, is elevating and comforting. Some even say that it is notorious for its aphrodisiac effects. Regardless, it makes for a very fragrant soap, with hints of nut and honey.

Ingredients:

INGREDIENTS FOR BASIC VEGETABLE SOAP

4 OUNCES BEESWAX

2 TABLESPOONS FINELY GROUND ALMONDS

1 TEASPOON FINELY GROUND CINNAMON

1 OUNCE SWEET ALMOND OIL

1 OUNCE HONEY (SLIGHTLY WARMED)

1 OUNCE NUTMEG ESSENTIAL OIL

- Follow instructions for Basic Vegetable Soap, adding beeswax to oils and vegetable shortening so that they heat up and melt together before blending them with the water–lye solution.

- Just after the soap mixture has started tracing, quickly add essential oil, sweet almond oil, ground almonds, honey and cinnamon. Stir until all ingredients are well blended. Pour mixture into greased molds and cover with a blanket or towel.

- Follow aging and drying instructions (see Sitting, Cooling and Aging).

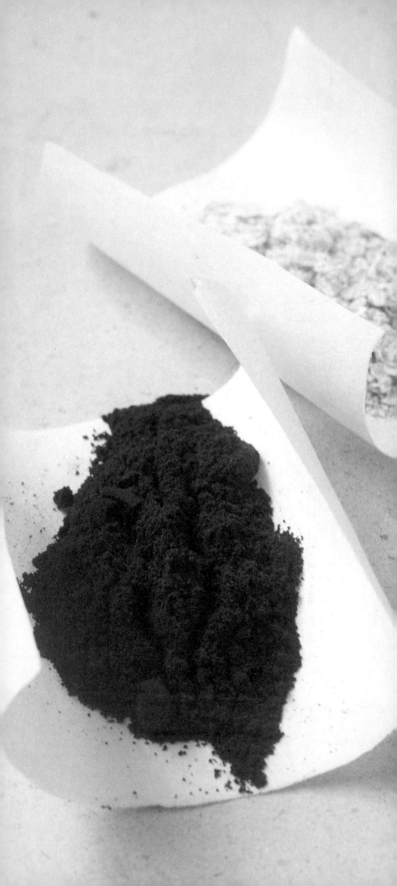

All-Purpose Coffee Oatmeal Soap

The combination of coffee and oatmeal makes this an ideal soap to have in the kitchen. Ground coffee gives this soap a rich, brown speckled color and wonderful aroma. It will also help rid hands of any strong cooking smells (such as onions or fish). Oatmeal will gently soften overworked and irritated skin. Although this recipes calls for the Basic Animal Fat soap recipe to yield a harder and longer lasting bar, it can also be duplicated using the Basic Vegetable Soap recipe for a softer bar with a frothier lather.

Ingredients:

INGREDIENTS FOR BASIC ANIMAL FAT SOAP

4 TABLESPOONS FINELY GROUND
COFFEE BEANS

4 TABLESPOONS OF FINELY GROUND OATMEAL

- Follow instructions for Basic Animal Fat Soap.

- Just after soap mixture has started to trace, add ground coffee beans and oatmeal.

- Stir until thoroughly blended and pour into molds. Follow aging and drying instructions (see Sitting, Cooling and Aging).

WHEN USING ANIMAL FAT, IT MUST BE FREE FROM DIRT, SALT, AND OTHER IMPURITIES. IT MUST ALSO BE FRESH OR IT WILL GIVE THE FINISHED PRODUCT A VERY UNPLEASANT RANCID ODOR.

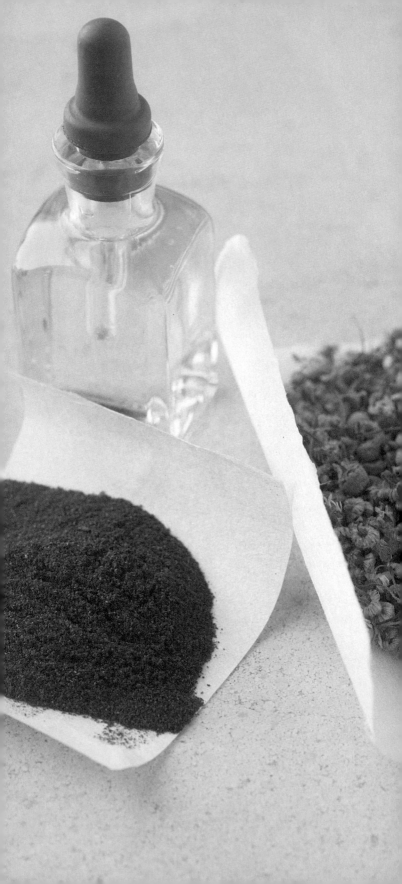

Chamomile and Sweet Almond Oil Soap

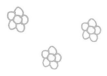

Dried chamomile promotes relaxation and calm. In soap, it helps heal dry and sensitive skin and serves as a gentle astringent. The sweet almond oil enhances the barís moisturizing properties. An ideal soap to bring in the bath.

Ingredients:

INGREDIENTS FOR BASIC VEGETABLE SOAP

2 OUNCES SWEET ALMOND OIL

2 OUNCES DRIED CHAMOMILE FLOWERS

1 OUNCE CHAMOMILE ESSENTIAL OIL

1 TEASPOON PAPRIKA (FOR COLOR)

- Follow instructions for Basic Vegetable Soap, page 64.

- Just after soap mixture has started to trace, add sweet almond oil and chamomile essential oil and blend thoroughly.

- Gradually add in dried chamomile flowers and paprika while stirring. Pour into molds .

- Follow aging and drying instructions (see Sitting, Cooling and Aging).

WHEN MAKING HERBAL SOAPS, YOU CAN REPLACE
THE WATER IN THE RECIPE WITH HERB TEA.

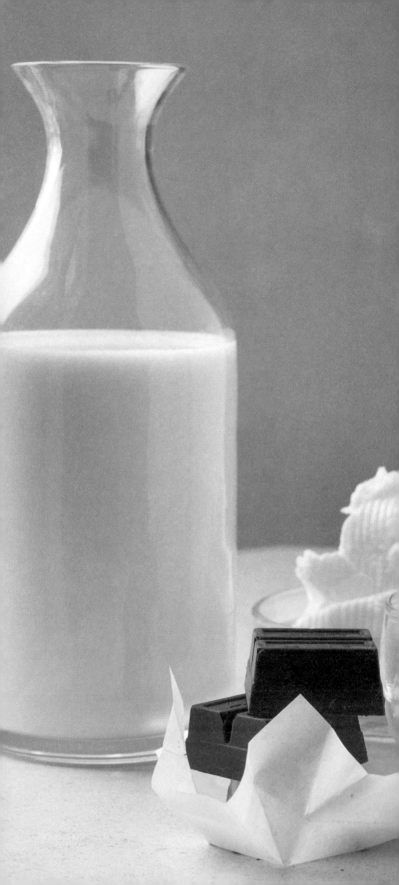

Chocolate Milk Soap

A chocoholic's dream come true. Baking chocolate will give this bar a creamy light brown color and an enticing aroma that will make kids—and adults—never want to get out of the bathtub!

Ingredients:

INGREDIENTS FOR BASIC ANIMAL FAT SOAP, BUT
REDUCE THE AMOUNT OF WATER TO 14 OUNCES
(INSTEAD OF 16 OUNCES)
1 / 2 OUNCE BAKING CHOCOLATE
2 OUNCES MILK
(COW'S MILK, GOAT'S MILK, BUTTERMILK)

- Follow instructions for Basic Animal Fat Soap, melting chocolate with animal fat, and combining milk and water before adding lye.

- Pour into molds.

- Follow aging and drying instructions (see Sitting, Cooling and Aging).

IF YOU WANT YOUR SOAP TO FLOAT,
FOLD AIR INTO THE SOAP MIXTURE WHEN IT IS THICK
ENOUGH BUT BEFORE POURING IT INTO MOLDS.

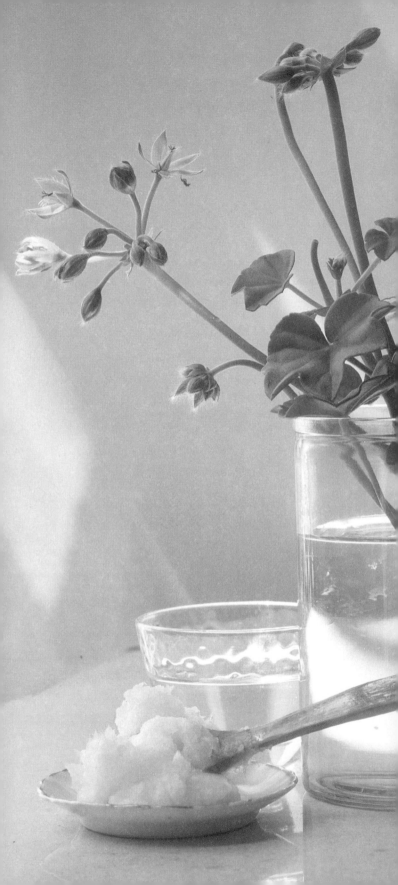

Indulging Geranium and Cocoa Butter Soap

Cocoa butter, which is extracted from the seeds of the cacao tree, is a rich emollient that softens and protects skin. It also enhances the texture of the bar by making it harder and creamy. Avocado oil, which contains large amounts of vitamins A, D and E, as well as amino acids and proteins, is an effective skin moisturizer and healer. Geranium essential oil has a slightly sweet rosy, lemon and mint smell that is very calming. The petals add unique color and texture to the bar.

Ingredients:

INGREDIENTS FOR BASIC VEGETABLE SOAP

2 OUNCES OF COCOA BUTTER

1 OUNCE GERANIUM ESSENTIAL OIL

1 TABLESPOON DRIED GERANIUM PETALS

1 OUNCE AVOCADO OIL

- Follow instructions for Basic Vegetable Soap, page 64, adding avocado oil and cocoa butter to fats and heat them together, before blending with lye–water mixture.

- Just as soap mixture begins to trace, stir in geranium petals and geranium essential oil and blend thoroughly.

- Follow aging and drying instructions (see Sitting, Cooling and Aging).

COLORED SOAP WILL LIGHTEN IN COLOR
AS IT SETS AND COOLS.

Restoring Olive Oil Glycerin Soap with Vodka

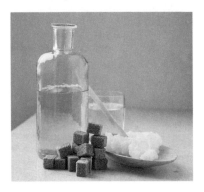

Glycerin is an emollient which exists naturally in vegetable and animal fats. This soap is particularly easy and quick to make. Once the glycerin is melted you can add essential oils, dried flowers, herbs, spices and dye without worrying about any adverse effects on the soap. The sugar and vodka render the soap transparent, which makes it more fun when adding trinkets, herbs or spices to the soap.

Ingredients:

14 OUNCES TALLOW

8 OUNCES COCONUT OIL

6 OUNCES OLIVE OIL

4 OUNCES PALM OIL

11 OUNCES WATER, PREFERABLY DISTILLED
AND AT ROOM TEMPERATURE

4 1/2 OUNCES LYE

1 OUNCE ESSENTIAL OIL OF CHOICE

Ingredients for added transparency:

2 OUNCES SUGAR

3 OUNCES WATER, PREFERABLY DISTILLED
AND AT ROOM TEMPERATURE

2 OUNCES GLYCERIN

4 OUNCES VODKA

- Place tallow and oils (with the exception of the essential oil) in a large lye resistant pot and heat until temperature is within 120°F to 135°F. Remove from heat.

- Measure out 11 ounces of water and put in a lye resistant pitcher with a pourable spout. Measure out lye and slowly add to water. Stir until lye is fully dissolved and temperature is within 120°F to135°F range (within the same temperature range as the oil mixture).

- Slowly add lye–water mixture to fat–oil mixture and stir regularly for about 20 to 25 minutes until tracing begins to occur. Blend in essential oil and pour into greased molds. Cover molds with a blanket or towels and place in a draft-free area for 24 hours, or until soap is firm to the touch.

- Take soap out of molds, cut into pieces and allow to age, uncovered and in a draft-free area for another two weeks.

- Place sugar in a bowl and set aside. Finely grate 8 ounces of the finished soap and slowly melt in a double boiler (or bowl placed over boiling water). Slowly add 2 ounces (leaving 1 ounce) of water, sugar and glycerin. Stir regularly until soap begins to thicken. Slowly add vodka and continue to stir over low heat.

- Add 1 ounce of heated water to sugar in bowl and stir until dissolved. Add sugar–water mixture to soap and continue to stir for about 35 minutes until soap begins to thicken. Pour soap into molds and place in freezer for 1 hour. Remove from freezer, take out of molds and place on a drying rack, piece of wax paper or plastic wrap and store in a draft-free area for two weeks.

- Your soap is now ready to be enjoyed!

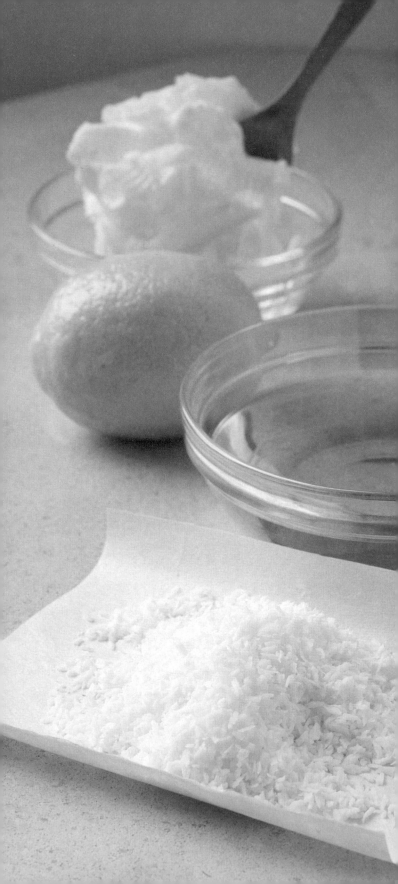

Lemon Lime Coconut Hair Bar

Once you have tried a hair bar, there is no going back to liquid shampoo. This particular bar is ideal for fine and delicate hair. The citrus oils cleanse the hair shaft and olive oil provides softness, shine and lather, while the egg yolk nourishes it. The lemon and lime will leave your hair smelling incredibly fresh.

Ingredients:

30 OUNCES OLIVE OIL

2 TABLESPOONS COCONUT OIL

2 OUNCES BEESWAX

1 EGG YOLK

1 OUNCE LIME ESSENTIAL OIL

1 OUNCE LEMON ESSENTIAL OIL

2 TABLESPOONS FINELY GRATED COCONUT

14 OUNCES OF WATER

4 1/2 OUNCES OF LYE

- Measure out 1 ounce of the olive oil and set aside the rest. Beat egg yolk into the 1 ounce of olive oil. In a lye and heat resistant pot, melt beeswax, olive oil (29 ounces), and coconut oil. Gradually stir in grated coconut. When temperature reaches between 120°F and 135°F , remove from heat.
- Measure out water and pour into a lye resistant pitcher with a pourable spout. Measure out lye and slowly add to water, stirring frequently until lye is fully dissolved.
- When lye/water mixture is within same temperature range as oils (120°F to 135°F) gently pour it into the oils until soap begins to trace (about 30 minutes). Whisk in olive oil–egg yolk mixture and blend thoroughly. Add lemon and lime essential oils, pour into molds, cover with a blanket or towel and set aside in a draft-free area for 24 hours or until firm to the touch. Remove from molds, place on a drying rack, and cut soap into bars. Store, uncovered in a draft-free area for four weeks.

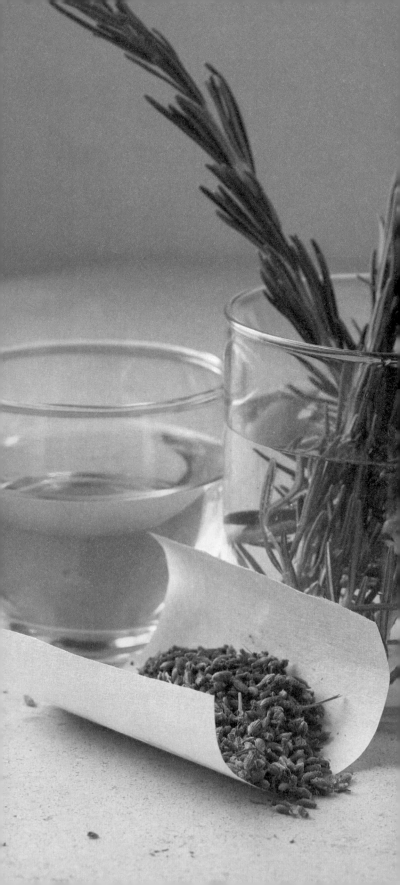

Rosemary Lavender Hair Bar

Rosemary essential oil is known for its ability to deep-cleanse and to soothe, especially headaches and chronic fatigue. The oil penetrates the scalp and promotes circulation and invigorates. Lavender, valued for its antiseptic and antibacterial properties, guarantees the bar's fragrant appeal. Jojoba and sweet almond oils are both excellent conditioners. This soap can be used as a shampoo bar and as a body bar.

Ingredients:

10 OUNCES COCONUT OIL

20 OUNCES OLIVE OIL

4 OUNCES SWEET ALMOND OIL

4 OUNCES JOJOBA OIL

16 OUNCES WATER, PREFERABLY DISTILLED
AND AT ROOM TEMPERATURE

5 1/2 OUNCES LYE

1 OUNCE LAVENDER ESSENTIAL OIL

1 OUNCE ROSEMARY ESSENTIAL OIL

- Follow instructions for Basic Vegetable Soap. Just as soap begins to trace, add lavender and rosemary essential oils.

- Follow aging and drying instructions (see Sitting, Cooling and Aging).

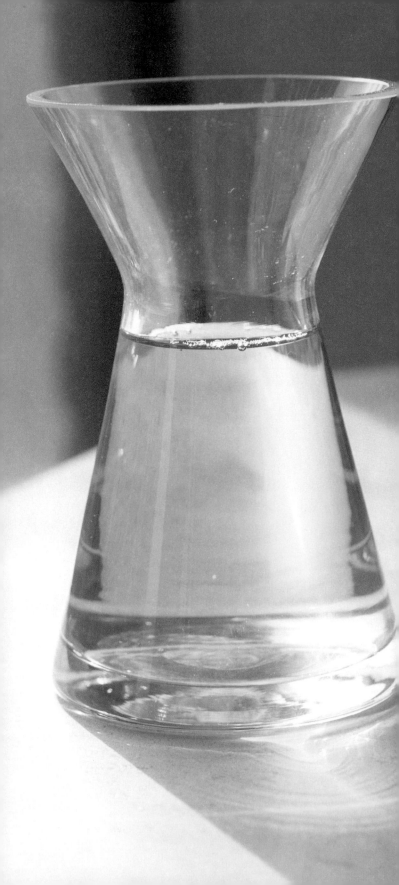

Hair Rinse

These rinses are incredibly simple to make and are highly effective for restoring the hair's natural pH balance and removing all residue form the hair shaft which could make it look dull, flat and lifeless. Use a rinse once a week, after conditioning hair, and rinse thoroughly with cool water.

Apple Cider Rinse

Ingredients:

2 OUNCES OF APPLE CIDER VINEGAR

8 OUNCES OF WATER

- *In a small bowl or jar, mix apple cider vinegar with water.*

SLOWLY POUR RINSE ONTO FRESHLY SHAMPOOED AND CONDITIONED HAIR. MAKE SURE TO KEEP YOUR EYES SHUT AS THE HIGH LEVEL OF ACIDITY WILL STING. RINSE THOROUGHLY. END WITH AS COOL A WATER RINSE AS YOU CAN STAND.

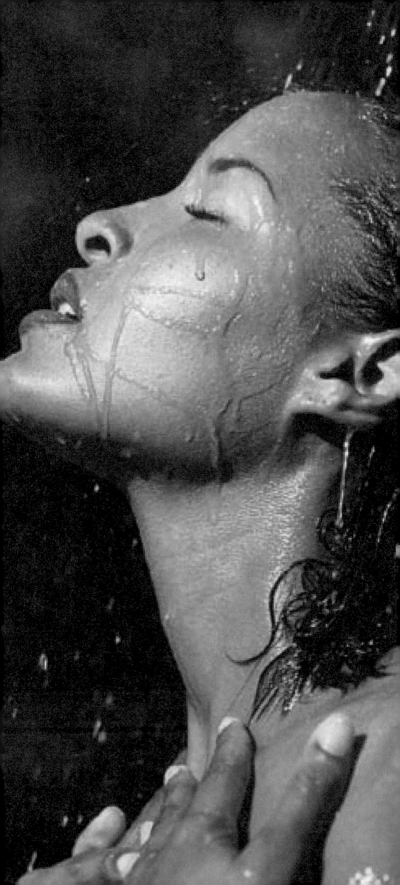

Parsely Lemon Rinse

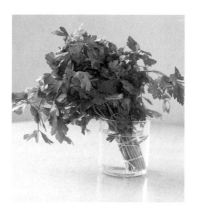

Ingredients:

THE JUICE OF ONE LEMON

2 OUNCES OF FINELY CHOPPED PARSLEY

(FOR ADDED SHINE)

8 OUNCES OF WATER

- *Bring 8 ounces of water to a boil, add parsley, and let stand for 5 minutes. Strain.*

- *Add lemon juice to parsley and water and allow to cool.*

SLOWLY POUR RINSE ONTO FRESHLY SHAMPOOED
AND CONDITIONED HAIR. MAKE SURE TO KEEP YOUR
EYES SHUT AS THE HIGH LEVEL OF ACIDITY WILL
STING. RINSE THOROUGHLY. END WITH AS COOL
A WATER RINSE AS YOU CAN STAND.

Even the most precise soapmaker may run into problems during the process or unexpected results at the finish. As you become more familiar with the elements of soapmaking, you will be able to identify problems before it is too late. Here are some common problems that just might crop up—and what to do if things don't seem quite right.

The soap won't come out of the mold:

- If you are having problems getting the soap out of the mold, put it in the freezer for an hour or so. The soap will "sweat" (the water in the soap migrates to the surface) and slide right out. See page 43 for greasing and lining molds.

Tracing does not occur:

- If your measurements were correct, tracing should occur—eventually. Be patient and keep stirring. If there is still no sign of tracing after one hour and a half, then there is a problem with the mixture (probably not enough lye or too much water). In this case, discard it and start a fresh batch.

The soap mixture is grainy:

- Grainy soap indicates that the temperatures were off at some point during the process or that the stirring was not brisk or regular enough. Nevertheless, the graininess is harmless and the soap can be used.

Air bubbles in the hardened soap:

- Bubbles are a result of stirring too briskly. Unfortunately, they often contain a liquid highly concentrated in lye. Make sure the bubbles are filled with air and not lye. If it is just air, the soap is perfectly fine—and chances are, it will float.

Large bright white chunks or pieces appear in the hardened soap:

- If too much lye was used in the process or stirring was too slow and insufficient, lye chunks will form in the soap. Discard this batch and start fresh.

When still in its liquid stage, the soap mixture looks like cottage cheese:

- This effect is known as "curdling," a result of inaccurate soap measurements, too much lye or a too rapid cooling stage. Although there are ways to save the soap, especially if the curdling is a result of an overly rapid cooling process, save yourself the headache and toss the batch.

The hardened soap smells bad:

- If your soap has an offensive smell to it, you have probably used too much animal fat or the fat itself was not fresh. The rancid odor will not go away and will only get worse with age. If you really can't stand the smell, throw the soap away.

The oil separates from the rest of the liquid after you've poured the soap:

- Separation indicates that either your measurements were off, there was a mistake in the soap-making process or there is too much lye in the soap mixture. Either way, throw the mixture away and start fresh.

A thin layer of oil or greasy substance appears on the surface of the soap after it has started to harden:

- Usually this is a result of the added essential oils which have risen to the surface. The essential oils will dissolve after the soap has fully set.

The soap is brittle, cracked and dry after it has set:

- Either the soap set too quickly and the cooling process was too fast (make sure you cover the soap with blankets or towels right after you have poured it into the molds), there was too much stirring during the soap-making process or there was too much lye in the mixture. Check your measurements.

The soap won't set:

- If after a few days the soap doesn't harden, there is probably too much water in the mixture, or not enough lye. Be patient and leave it in the mold. If your measurements were accurate, the soap will eventually harden. Remember: Soap made out of vegetable oil tends to stay softer than soap made out of animal fats.

The soap is streaked:

- Streaking indicates that the soap mixture was not stirred enough during saponification. It is harmless and the soap is completely usable.

White powder appears on the surface
of your soap after it has dried:

- This powder, caused by the contact between curing soap and air, is called "soda ash" and is harmless. Either scrape or slice off the ash with a knife before packaging the soap. You can also wash it away under running water and set aside to dry. Avoid or minimize ash altogether by placing plastic wrap or heavy duty wax paper over the soap mixture immediately after having poured it into the molds, and pressing it against the surface of the soap.

SOAP FACTS

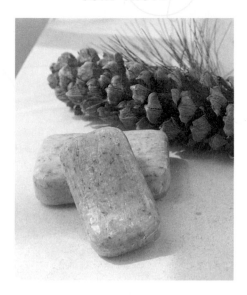

- The word soap comes from Mount Sapo where animals were sacrificed and the rain washed a mixture of animal fats and wood ashes into a sudsy component.

- During the 8th century, Italians and Spaniards used a substance made out of goat's fat and wood ashes, similar to soap.

- The English began soap–crafting during the 12th century.

- When radio programs were first broadcast in North America, product manufacturers saw this as a tremendous method by which to advertise their products. Major soap companies quickly seized the opportunity and began sponsoring radio programs that aired mostly during the day and whose prime audience were house-wives. Hence, soap operas.

- There is evidence of a soap factory and soap bars in the ruins of Pompeii in Rome.

- Early Greeks and Romans rubbed their bodies with sand and olive to clean themselves.

- Detergents differ from soaps in that they are made from petrole-um distillates, not fats or oils.

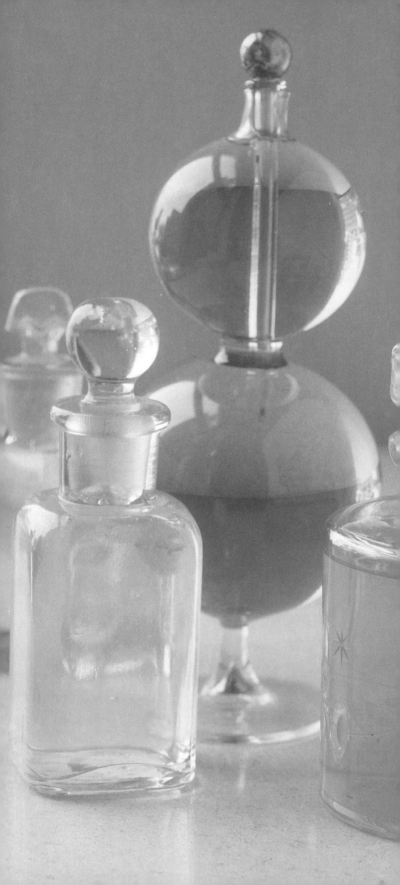

PART II

Making Scents

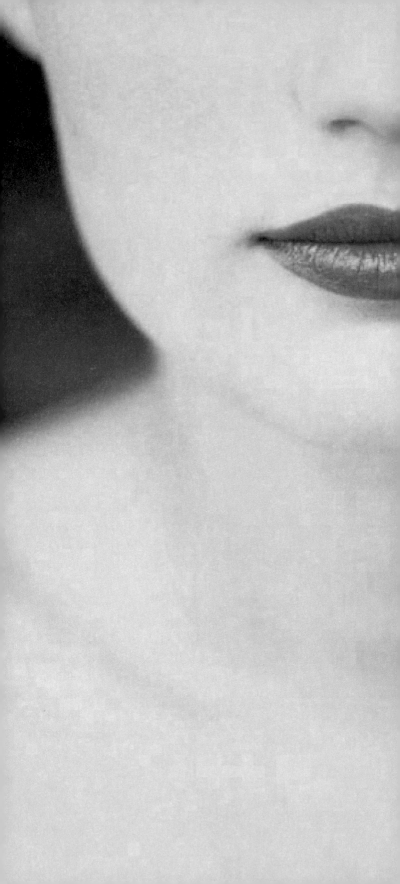

A Fragrant History

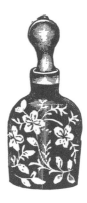

Perfume, as an art and concept, has been permeating our senses for many centuries. Aromatic artifacts dating as far back as 3500 BC provide many insights into the role fragrance has played in ancient civilizations. Whether used for scenting food, in the process of embalming and mummification, for medicinal purposes, or for carrying messages to the deities, perfume has had a tremendous impact on humanity. It has facilitated the expression of spirituality and religion, broadened economic trade (most of the raw materials, aromatic spices and herbs, were imported from Arabia, Persia, China and India) and reportedly rocked empires through its seductive nature.

The word perfume comes from *per fumum*, a Latin phrase which means "through smoke". In ancient Egypt, an incense known as kyphi was a sacred perfume burned in temples at sunset and in homes at night. This particular incense was a paste-like substance made from various gums and resins, aromatic herbs, honey, wine and raisins.

Although the Egyptians—and later the Greeks and Romans—were the first to use fragrances and oils for personal hygiene by rubbing them into moist skin after bathing, the Arabs were instrumental, especially during the Golden Age of Arabian civilization (8th to 10th centuries AD), in developing sophisticated techniques of distillation and perfume-making. They also successfully introduced unorthodox blends in which fruits, flowers and herbs were incorporated into animal perfumes such as musk, ambergris and civet. But it was not truly until the Renaissance that the use of fragrance as a way to express moods and evoke certain behavioral responses developed.

In the late 1300s, the very first alcohol-based fragrance, the pre-

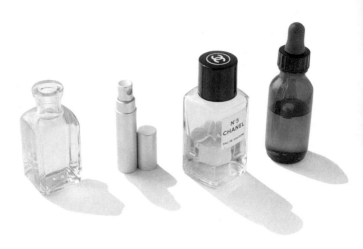

cursor of perfume as we know it today, made its debut. Hungary Water, created for Queen Elizabeth of Hungary, was in fact one of the earliest toilet waters ever made, and its recipe is still duplicated with slight variations for today's woman. The original Hungary Water contained rosemary, marjoram and pennyroyal distilled in wine alcohol. It is said to have been a key contribution to Queen Elizabeth's notorious beauty and youthful ways.

During the 16th century, the fragrance industry took another giant step forward with the advent of fine quality scented gloves. Scented leather gloves, popular in Spain and Portugal, became the fashion accessory of choice among the nobility in Europe. The gloves, perfumed by tanners to mask the unpleasant odor of natural hide, also came in handy as a way to combat unpleasant sanitation odors. The glove wearer would simply hold up the scented glove to the nose, and take a whiff when crossing malodorous areas. In the 1530s, Catherine de Medici, for whom one of the oldest colognes was made by Florentine Dominicans, was responsible for introducing these scented gloves to France. She was instrumental in establishing a laboratory solely for the study of perfume in Grasse, a town in Provence, the South of France.

Known today as the workroom of the fragrance industry, Grasse was originally famed for its tanneries. In fact, until the late 1700s, perfume makers in France were simultaneously Glovers and Perfumers. Gradually, as leather goods became less popular, many tanners gave up working with hide to focus solely on manufacturing fragrances. Today, Grasse continues to be home to over 35 factories that process perfume materials, and is considered by many the fragrance capital of the world. Its mild climate and geographical location make it an ideal heaven for flower and plant growing.

By the 18th century, perfume had permeated the walls of French aristocracy. Versailles literally bathed in perfume as its ruler, Louis XIV took on the surname of Le Roi Parfum (the Perfume King). His mood notoriously dictated the court's perfume of the day. And often, dousing oneself with perfume was a preferred alternative to bathing.

But because of the high cost of imported raw materials and amount required to produce a particular fragrance, perfume remained a luxury item, reserved exclusively for the nobility.

It's not until the late 1800's when the first synthetic fragrances were manufactured, thus bypassing the prohibitive expense of natural raw materials, that perfume became accessible to a wider range of people.

Today, the fragrance industry is a billion-dollar one. It has infiltrated multiple aspects of our daily lives: from perfumes, colognes, soaps and hair products, to fabric softeners, deodorants and food. It leaps from the pages of magazines, helps define a fashion designer's personae and adds mystique and character to anyone who uses it. It is an expression of individuality, yet remains a reassuring constant by evoking familiar situations and emotions. Fragrance transports us through space and transcends time.

However you choose to fragrance your world and whatever you choose to do it with, never underestimate the power and lure of scent. Cleopatra conquered emperors with it. Napoleon wouldn't go into battle without having at least one flask of it on hand.

As Coco Chanel once said, "Elegance is not possible without fragrance."

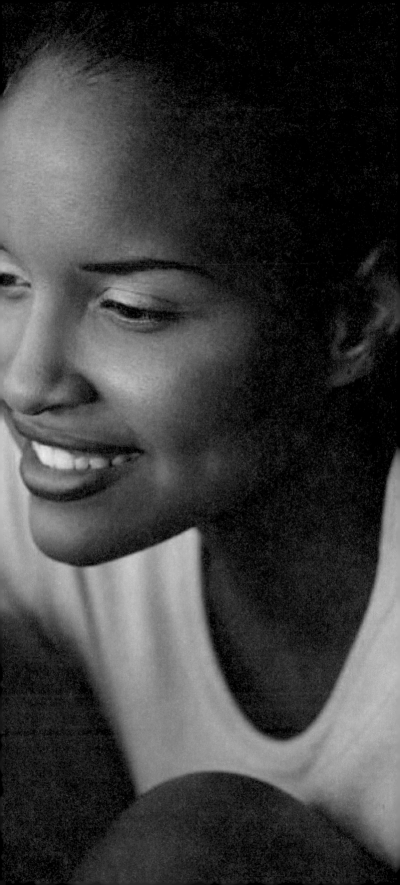

FRAGRANCE FAMILIES

Fragrances are divided into families, each with its own specific character and scent: Floral, Green, Modern/Aldehydic, Chypre, Oriental/Amber, Citrus, Spicy and Oceanic.

When you've selected the fragrance family (or families) that work best for you, it's important to consider the following factors: personal preference, lifestyle, mood and your skin's chemical reaction to a fragrance. Remember that a perfume that smells one way on one individual will most likely smell different on another.

When trying out fragrances, it's best to choose one of lighter concentration such as eau de cologne, and dab it sparingly on the wrist area. Leave it to air dry for 45 minutes to an hour, so there is enough time to let all the different notes have a chance to surface. (See How to Read a Fragrance, page 126.)

Floral

Floral is by far the largest of the fragrance families. A little over half of all the brand name perfumes on the market today fall into this category. Floral fragrances contain primarily essential oils from flowers and can be divided into four subcategories: floral, floral/sweet, floral/fresh, and floral/fruity/fresh. Scents include rose, lily of the valley, marigold, narcissus, magnolia, honeysuckle, gardenia, orchid, geranium, sweet pea, violets, orange blossoms, jasmine and tuberose.

WEARER/MOOD PROFILE:
Feminine, delicate and romantic

WHEN TO WEAR IT:
Ideal for daytime wear and summer evenings

Examples:
SUBLIME (JEAN PATOU)
VIVID (LIZ CLAIBORNE)
DUNE (CHRISTIAN DIOR)
360 DEGREES (PERRY ELLIS)
TRESOR (LANCOME)
SAFARI (RALPH LAUREN)
L'AIR DU TEMPS (NINA RICCI)
VERSUS (VERSACE PROFUMI)
GIORGIO (GIORGIO BEVERLY HILLS)
DKNY (DONNA KARAN)
CHANEL N^O 22 (CHANEL)
ANAIS ANAIS (CACHAREL)
TRIBU (BENETTON)
POISON (CHRISTIAN DIOR)
JOY (JEAN PATOU)
ANNE KLEIN (ANNE KLEIN)
BEAUTIFUL (ESTEE LAUDER)

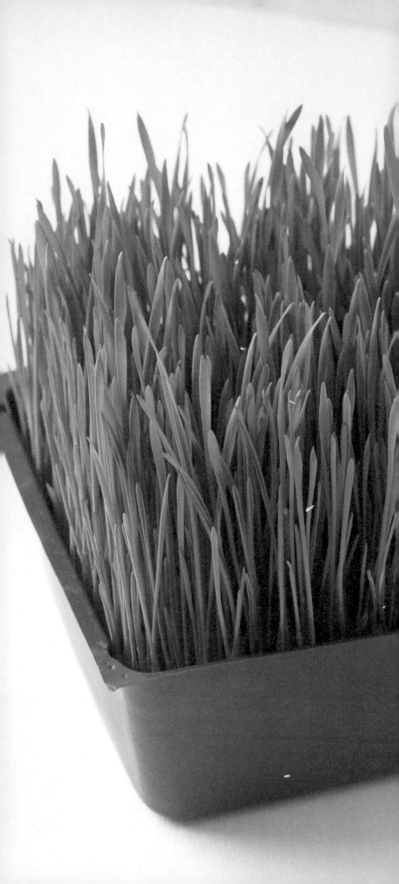

FRAGRANCE FAMILIES

Green

These fragrances evoke the smell of freshly mowed grass, summer meadows, new spring leaves and crisp pine. They are a combination of herbal blends, plant greens, citrus and moss. Green notes are natural in character, often married with fruity and floral notes.

Wearer/Mood Profile:
SPORTY, SPIRITED, SOCIAL, LIVELY,
ENERGETIC, OUTGOING,
MODERN AND FASHIONABLE

When to wear it:
DAYTIME AND CASUAL SUMMER EVENINGS

Examples:
ALLIAGE (ESTEE LAUDER)
VENT VERT (BALMAIN)
AMORENA (CANTILÈNE)
CHANEL N° 19 (CHANEL)
DRAKKAR (LAROCHE)
EAU DE FRAICHEUR (WEIL)
JIL SANDER (SANDER)
MADEMOISELLE RICCI (NINA RICCI)
SILENCES (JACOMO)
SILVERLINE (GAINSBOROUGH)
SPORT SCENT FOR WOMEN (JOVAN)

Modern/Aldehydic

As their name suggests, these fragrances are derived from aldehydes, a chemical group of compounds which were discovered in the late 1800s, and that were put to use in the perfume industry by Ernest Beaux, the perfumer who created the first aldehydic perfume, Chanel N° 5. Essentially, aldehydes are aroma chemicals which play against each other and with natural aromas to create a final fragrance. Most of the perfumes manufactured today contain aldehydes.

Wearer Mood/Profile:

RADIANT, ORIGINAL, SPIRITED

When to wear it:

DAYTIME WEAR OR EVENING

Examples:

CHANEL N° 5 (CHANEL)

WHITE DIAMONDS (ELIZABETH TAYLOR)

RED (GIORGIO BEVERLY HILLS)

MADAME ROCHAS (ROCHAS)

ESCAPE (CALVIN KLEIN)

CLAIBORNE (LIZ CLAIBORNE)

ARPEGE (LANVIN)

ANTILOPE (WEIL)

BAGHARI (PIGUET)

AVIANCE (MATCHABELLI)

CALINE (JENA PATOU)

CAPRICCI (NINA RICCI)

CHICANE (JACOMO)

CHANTAGE (LANCASTER)

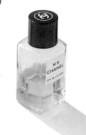

Chypre

Named after a perfume made in Cyprus that was famous during Roman times, these fragrances are based on oak moss, patchouli, civet, labdanum, musk and clary sage, with occasional citrus and floral traces. They are rich and tenacious in character.

Wearer/Mood Profile:
ELEGANT, FORMAL, SOPHISTICATED

When to wear it:
BEST FOR EVENING WEAR

Examples:
CABOCHARD (GRÈS)

MA GRIFFE (CARVEN)

YSATIS (GIVENCHY)

HALSTON (HALSTON BORGHESE)

ANIMALE (SUZANNE DE LYON)

MISS DIOR (DIOR)

AMERIQUE (COURRÈGES)

BANDIT (PIGUET)

APHRODISIA (FABERGÉ)

BAT SHEBA (MULLER)

CACHET (MATCHABELLI)

CIALENGA (BALENICAGA)

CIAO (HOUBIGANT)

GRAIN DE PASSION (VERFAILLIE)

NUEVA MAJA (MYRURGIA)

NITCHEVO (JUVENA)

SCULPTURA (JOVAN)

SECRET DE VENUS (WEIF)

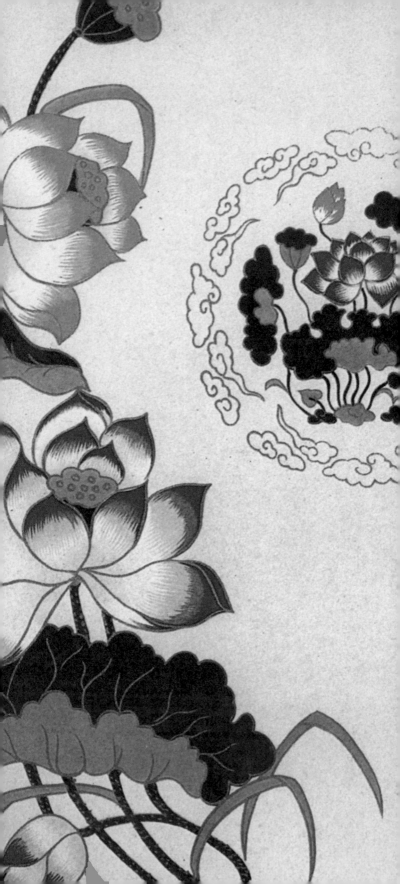

Fragrance Families

Amber/Oriental

This family evokes exotic spices and essences, leather, caramel and warmth. Oriental fragrances are heavy and have long staying power. Scents in this family include musks, amber, resins, deep woody smells and vanilla.

Wearer/Mood Profile:
MYSTERIOUS, SEDUCTIVE, FEMININE

When to wear it:
IDEAL FOR EVENING WEAR

Examples:
OBSESSION (CALVIN KLEIN)
NINJA (PARFUMS DE COEUR)
SHALIMAR (GUERLAIN)
INCOGNITO (COVER GIRL)
NAVY (COVER GIRL)
SAMSARA (GUERLAIN)
CHANTILLY (PARQUET)
OPIUM (YVES ST. LAURENT)
EMERAUDE (COTY)
BIJAN (BIJAN)
ASJA (FENDI)
KEORA (COUTURIER)
KL (LAGERFELD)

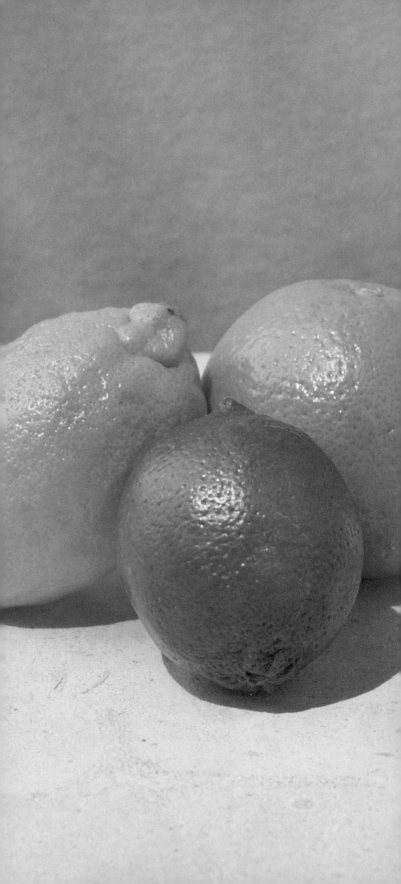

Citrus

Citrus fragrances are light, clean and fresh smelling and are best suited for eau de toilette. They include the scents of lemons, oranges,
limes, mandarins, cedrat, lemon grass, verbena and bergamot.

Wearer/Mood Profile:

YOUTHFUL, FEMININE

When to wear it:

IDEAL FOR DAYTIME OR
CASUAL SUMMER EVENINGS

Examples:

EAU D'HADRIEN (ANNICK GOUTAL)
EAU D'HERMÉS (HERMÉS)
EAU DE COLOGNE HERMÉS (HERMÉS)
EAU FRAICHE (DIOR)
E DE C DU COQ (GUERLAIN)
Ô DE LÂNCOME (LÂNCOME)

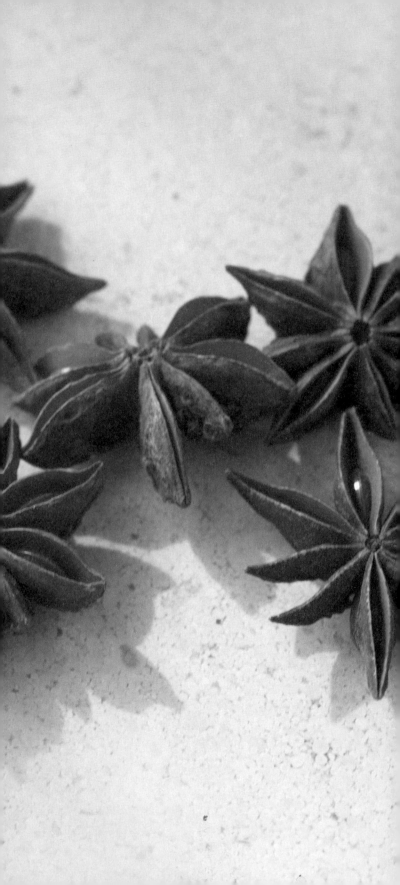

Spicy

Spicy fragrances have medium to long lasting power. Cinnamon, nutmeg, cassia, cloves, pimento and mace are a few of the scents included in this family.

Wearer/Mood Profile:
INNOVATIVE, ORIGINAL, OUTGOING,
SOCIAL, UNCONVENTIONAL

When to wear it:
EVENING

Examples:
CHALDEE (PATOU)
FLEURS D'ORLANE (ORLANE)
INDRA (ST PRES)
MA LIBERTE (PATOU)
MALMAISON (FLORIS)
MOODS (KRIZIA)
CINNABAR (ESTEE LAUDER)
MOMENT SUPREME (PATOU)
PARFUM SACRÉ (CARON)
POISON (DIOR)
NAHEMA (GUERLAIN)
TRANCE (BETRIX)

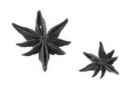

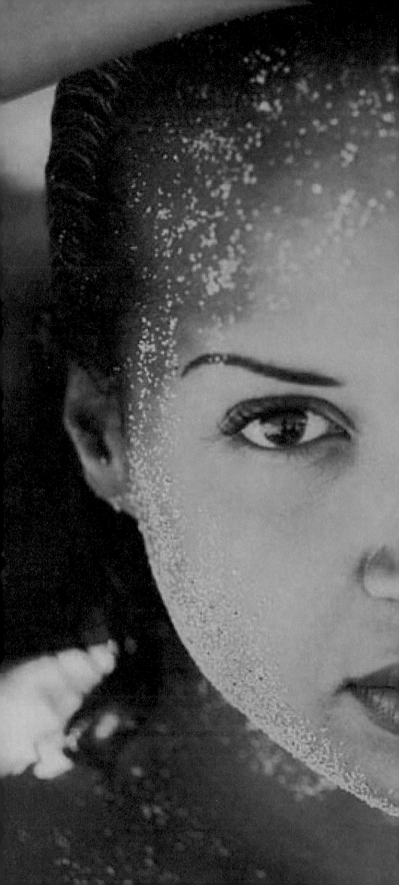

Oceanic

This is a recent addition to the fragrance families. Oceanic fragrances are made up entirely of synthetic materials. Oceanic fragrance aromas are chemically created to simulate the smell of freshly cleaned linens, ocean breeze, clean mountain air and lakeside picnics.

Wearer/Mood Profile:

OUTDOORSY, ATHLETIC,
INDEPENDENT, ENERGETIC

When to wear it:

IDEAL FOR DAYWEAR
AND CASUAL SUMMER EVENING

Examples:

L'EAU D'ISSEY (ISSEY MIYAKE)
ACQUA DI GIO (ARMANI)
CRISTALLE (CHANEL)
DUNE (DIOR)
SUNFLOWERS (ARDEN)
WHITE LINEN (ESTEE LAUDER)

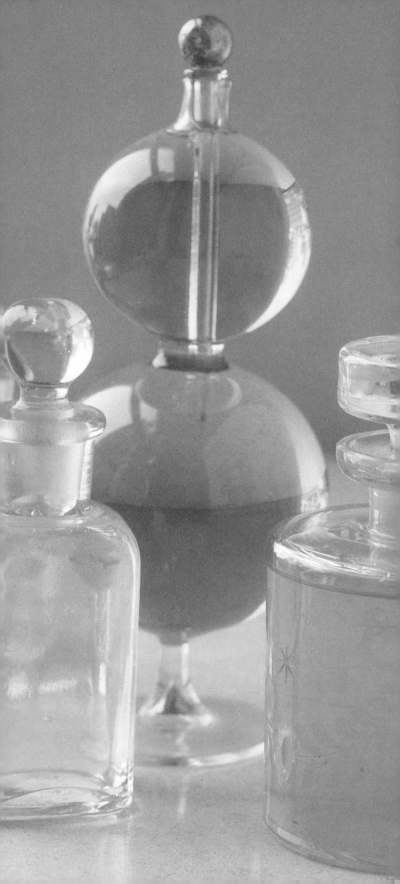

How to Read a Fragrance

There are essentially three types of fragrances: classical or classically structured fragrances, single note fragrances and linear fragrances. It is important to identify the fragrance type you're dealing with before making an attempt to read.

Classical Fragrances

Most perfumes on the market today fall into this type. These fragrances are elaborate mixtures of anywhere up to 700 ingredients, sometimes natural and sometimes synthetic, and are structured in three acts or movements. Like movements in a piece of classical music, they blend harmoniously—and sometimes imperceptibly—into each other.

The fragrance industry takes much of its terminology from music. Like music, perfume is composed of notes, each with a specific character, purpose and impact; each leaving a different impression over varying periods of time.

Classically structured fragrances are comprised of three distinct notes—top, middle and base—and each note lives out its own phase or lifespan. While an individual note has a specific identity, the collaboration and harmonious blending of all three notes, the smooth flow from one phase to the next, is what makes a fragrance work. In perfume terminology, this smooth flow is called an accord, and is precisely what a perfumer strives to achieve when creating a new fragrance.

Single note fragrances:

Single note fragrances focus on one specific scent. This scent, whether from a flower or plant for example, will often be mixed with other ingredients that will help intensify the primary note or scent and affect its duration. Prior to the introduction of classic fragrances at the end of the 19th century, most fragrances were single note ones and were composed primarily of essential oils like rose, or geranium.

Linear fragrances:

Unlike classic fragrances, linear fragrances as their name suggests are constant in how they smell. While they may have middle notes and bottom notes, they tend to have the same impact and impression four hours later as when they were first applied.

How to Read a Fragrance

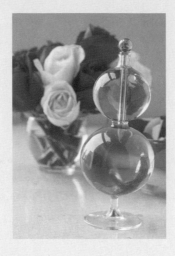

TOP NOTES (*also called head notes*) are responsible for the perfume's first impression. Top notes surface right after the perfume has been applied to the skin. These notes tend to be striking and impactful, but are also the most volatile: They only last a few minutes. After they have faded, phase two begins and the middle notes take center stage.

MIDDLE NOTES (*also called heart or medium notes*) constitute the 'meat' or the dominant trait of the perfume. They start to appear on the skin about ten minutes after the fragrance is first applied and can last up to several hours. In many ways, the middle notes determine the basic character or signature of a fragrance and will help classify the perfume into a fragrance family (see Fragrance Families, page 109). Middle notes dictate whether the fragrance is green, floral, spicy, oriental, chypre, modern or oceanic.

BASE NOTES (*also called lower notes or back notes*) are most discernible once the middle notes begin to fade. Base notes are responsible for the duration of a fragrance on the skin as well as its depth and intensity. They supply the perfume with fixatives, a natural or synthetic substance that can be animalic (a fragrant material of animal origin like musk, ambergris or civet), resinous (like balsam, galbanum and frankincense), or woody in nature (aloe wood, orris root, or tarragon leaves). Fixatives prolong the evaporation rate of a fragrance and makes other scents mixed with it last longer. Traces of base notes can last on the skin for hours, even sometimes a few days.

Notes

Top Notes:

FLORAL, FRUITY AND CITRUS:
*rose, marigold, iris, gardenia, geranium,
jasmine, lily of the valley, tuberose,
chamomile, peach, black currant, apricot,
orange, lime, lemon, lemon verbena,
mandarin, bergamot, tangerine*

SPICY:
*cinnamon, clove, pepper, nutmeg,
coriander, allspice*

WOODY:
sandalwood, rosemary, cedar, oakmoss

Rosemary

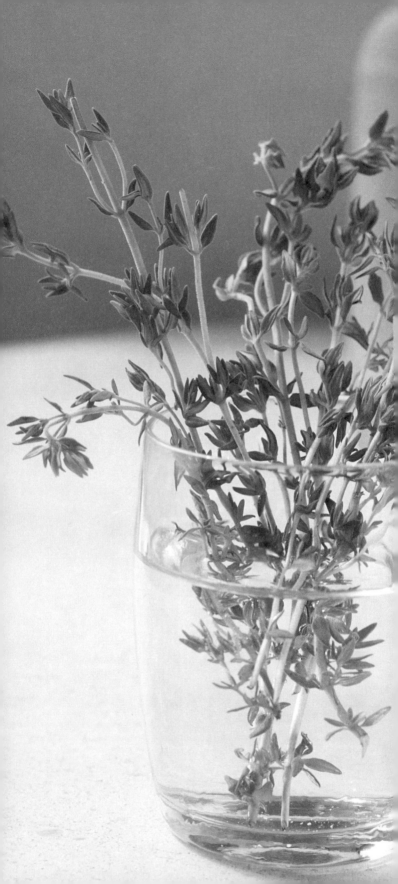

Middle Notes:

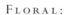

FLORAL:
rose, jasmine, orchid, lavender, iris, orange flower, geranium, camellia, lily of the valley, gardenia, tuberose, ylang-ylang

GREEN:
mostly aldehydes (aroma chemicals) which simulate the smell of freshly mowed grass and green leaves

MODERN:
aldehydes which simulate floral, fruity, citrus or woody notes Oriental/Amber: musk, amber, vanilla

CHYPRE:
storax, calamus, oak moss, patchouli, labdanum, clary sage

CITRUS:
lemon, lime, orange, lemon verbena, bergamot, pettitgrain, mandarin, tangerine

SPICY:
cinnamon, coriander, pepper, pimento, nutmeg, allspice, clove, ginger, myrrh

OCEANIC:
aldehydes which simulate the smell of freshly washed linens and sea air

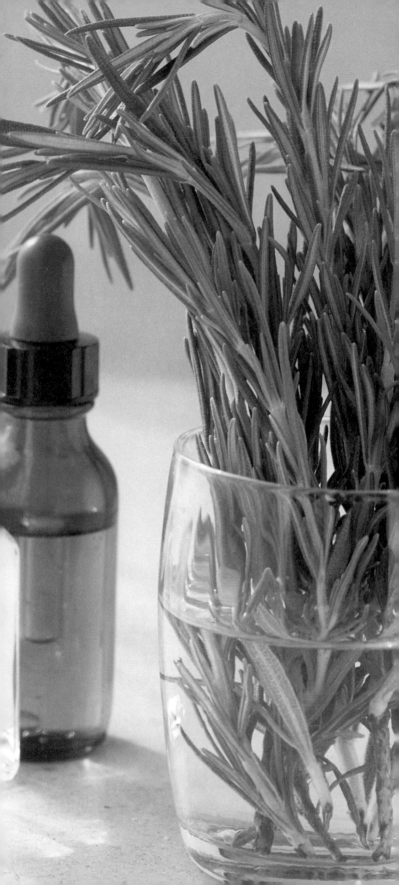

NOTES

Base Notes:

ANIMALIC:
civet, musk, ambergris, castoreum

RESINOUS:
balsam, angelica root, galbanum,
frankincense, Copaiba resin, balsam of Judea,
balm of Gilead, balm of Peru, Tolu balsam

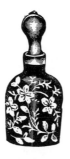

WOODY:
vetivert, oakmoss, patchouli, vanilla,
sandalwood, aloewood, ambrein, benzoin,
musk, orris root, tarragon leaves,
tonka, Virginia cedar, cedarwood

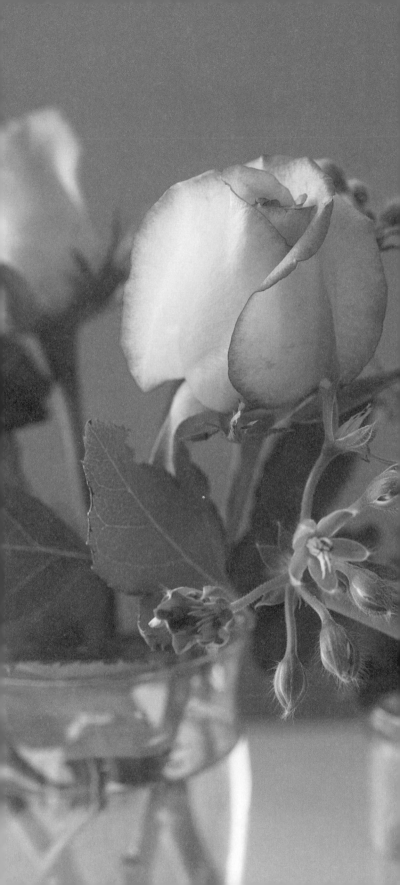

Perfume Recipes

ROSE WATER

•

LAVENDER WATER

•

SWEET ORANGE SPLASH

•

LEMON LIME COLOGNE

•

CLARY SAGE & THYME COLOGNE

•

OAKMOSS PERFUME BLEND

•

SPICE SPLASH

•

VANILLA BEAN WATER

•

PEAR NECTAR PERFUME

•

PROVENCE PERFUME OIL

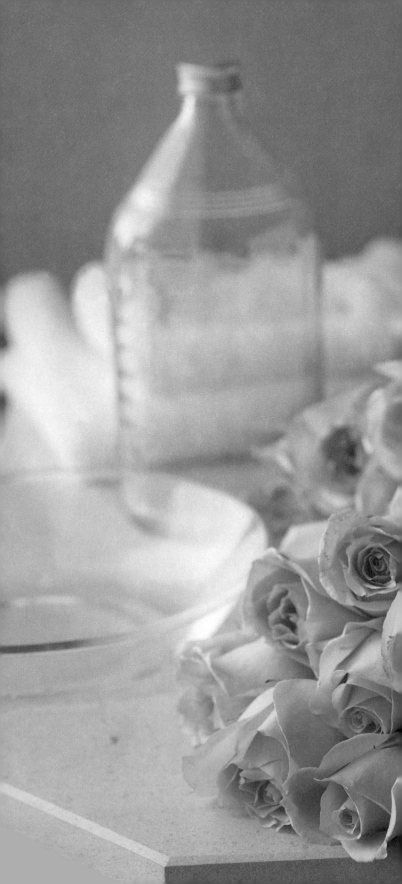

TOOLS OF THE TRADE

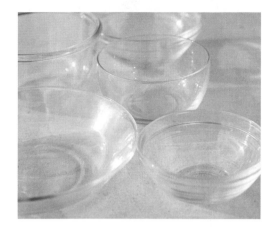

Very few tools are required for creating fragrances at home. In fact, most of them can be found right in your own kitchen, perhaps with the exception of small glass bottles in which to keep the final fragrance (see Resources, page 178)

- Glass containers with an airtight lid: A clean mayonnaise jar will do the trick. This jar is to mix and steep ingredients before pouring into decanters and bottles. Make sure they are clean and completely dry—preferably sterilized—before use.

- Glass stirring rod or stainless steel spoon: for stirring oils and ingredients.

- Measuring cups and spoons: for measuring water, oils, herbs, spices and flowers

- Droppers: for carefully measuring essential oils. Small funnel: for filling bottles and decanters; glass is preferable. Small amber (dark) glass bottles with stoppers or lids: for storing fragrances.

- Cheese cloth or paper coffee filter: for straining herbs, spices, and flowers out of liquids.

- Blotter paper: for testing scents.

- Distilled water

- 100 Proof Vodka

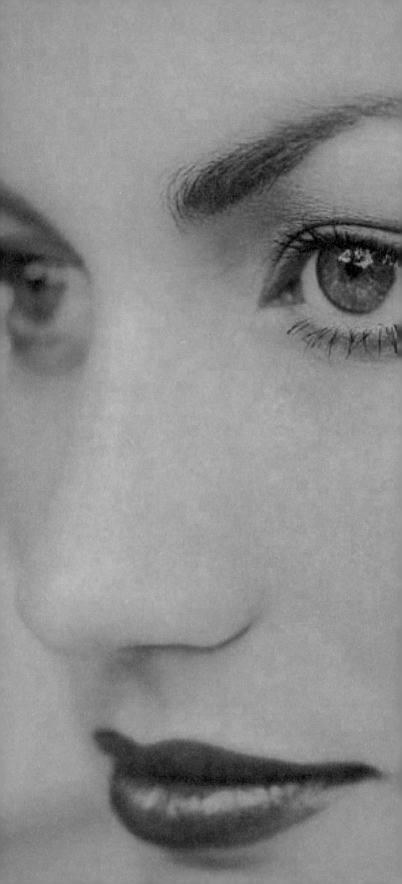

MAKING SCENTS

Making fragrances at home is not about trying to reproduce Chanel N$^{O.}$ 5 notes on the kitchen counter or concocting a version of L'Air du Temps in your basement. The creation of these perfumes is best left in the hands—and noses—of perfumers and perfume manufacturers who have the training, talent and access to materials and methods that even the most eager home fragrance creator would have a hard time duplicating.

Making scents at home is experimenting with and creating customized fragrances—sprays, essences, perfume oils, colognes and waters—that blend with and reflect personal emotions, moods and lifestyle. These scents are made with simple ingredients and tools that are now readily available through mail order, the Internet, health food stores, specialty shops and sometimes even the local grocer.

When one thinks of using fragrances, the first thing that comes to mind is dabbing a scent on the wrist, leaving a trace delicately behind the ear or subtly behind the arc of the knee. While the fragrances in this chapter are particularly suited for scenting the "self," their aromatic qualities can expand beyond the immediate entourage, and with a little creativity and imagination, will permeate all aspects of the home.

The following are a few simple recipes, with selections from the fragrance families (see page 109), with the exception of Modern/Aldehydic, Green and Oceanic fragrances, which can only be made in a laboratory due to the inorganic nature of their components. These sprays, splashes and colognes are exquisite on their own, or they can serve as a base for making other fragrances by adding additional ingredients such as fragrance oils, essential oils, herbs, spices and flowers.

NOTE: When crafting these fragrances, it is important to use the highest quality ingredients possible. Use 100-proof vodka and distilled or bottled water only; and fresh or dried herbs, flowers and fruits that were not colored or chemically treated.

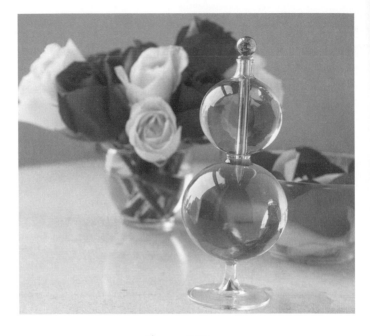

Rose Water

PROFILE

Fragrance Family: Floral
Single Note: Floral

The rose has played a variety of roles through history. There is evidence of its use as early as 600 BC. Wreaths made out of roses were found in ancient Egyptian tombs; the Romans filled pillows with rose petals; the Greeks dubbed the blossom "the Queen of Flowers"; and during the Middle Ages, roses acquired a medicinal use in addition to a religious one. The growing interest in the flower brought on the perfection of rose oil distillation, which came about in Persia in the 16th century. The Turks were responsible for introducing the process to Europe, which today remains one of the most prominent rose oil producers of the world.

Rose oil—also called rose attar or rose otto—continues to play center stage in the perfume industry. The most popular rose from which oil is extracted is the Damask Rose, one of the most ancient garden roses, introduced to Europe by early Arab perfume makers.

Approximately 75 percent of all quality perfumes on the market today list rose oil as one of their main ingredients. But since it takes approximately 10,000 pounds of roses to distill one pound of oil, rose attar remains an extremely costly fragrant, which is why synthetic fragrances are so often substituted. There are about as many different recipes for rose water as there are types of roses, of which there are over 1,000. This particular recipe is authentic and simple. The alcohol serves as a preservative and prolongs shelf life to up to six to eight months. If prepared without alcohol, rosewater should be used within one month.

Ingredients:

1 CUP DISTILLED WATER

2 1/2 TABLESPOONS VODKA

1/2 CUP FRESH ROSE PETALS

10 DROPS ROSE FRAGRANCE OIL

- *Fill a sterilized glass jar with rose petals.*

- *Pour water and vodka over petals, stirring gently with a glass rod or stainless steel spoon.*

- *Add rose fragrance oil and seal with an airtight lid.*

- *Store in a cool place for one week, and stir every few days.*

- *Strain liquid through cheese cloth or a paper filter and discard petals.*

- *Rose water should be bottled immediately in an airtight bottle.*

ROSE WATER WAS FIRST DISTILLED IN THE
11TH CENTURYBY AN ARABIAN DOCTOR AND CHEMIST.

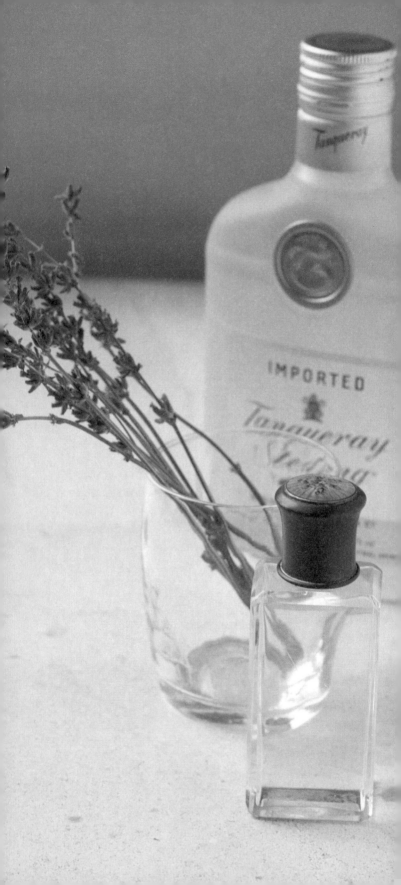

Lavender Water

PROFILE
Fragrance Family: Floral
Single Note: Floral

Lavender—which comes from the word "lavare," Latin for "to wash"—has been a favorite ingredient in perfume making since the ancient Greeks and Romans, who made much use of it in their bath water. It has a sweetly floral aroma with herbal and slight balsamic undertones. In addition to its fragrant powers, lavender is said to possess a multitude of healing properties: It is effective as an antiseptic or antibiotic, it prevents scarring, soothes burns and treats infections, helps regenerate skin cells and relieves muscle pain, headaches, fatigue, insomnia, depression and boosts immunity. Lavender water, which became popular in England in the 17th century, is soothing when used as a body splash. Apply by hand or spray to relieve aching legs, to relax, refresh and to steady emotions.

Ingredients:

1 CUP DISTILLED WATER

2 1/2 TABLESPOONS VODKA

10 DROPS LAVENDER ESSENTIAL OIL

1/2 CUP LAVENDER FLOWERS (FRESH OR DRIED)

- Fill a sterilized jar with lavender. Pour water and vodka over lavender and stir with a glass rod or stainless steel spoon.

- Add lavender essential oil, steal with an airtight lid and set in a cool, dark place for one week, stirring every few days.

- Strain liquid through cheese cloth or a paper filter and discard dried lavender. Bottle lavender water immediately. It can be stored in a dark bottle and kept for up to one year.

NATIVE TO PROVENCE, LAVENDER DATES BACK TO THE TIME OF ANCIENT ROME, WHEN ITS OIL WAS EXTRACTED AND USED AS AN ANTISEPTIC.

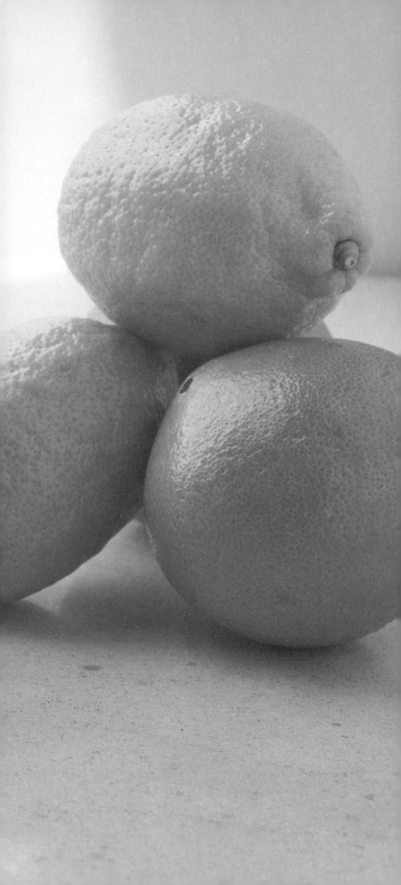

Sweet Orange Splash

PROFILE
Fragrance Family: Citrus
Single Note: Citrus

Orange, like other citrus oils, has a very volatile top note, but still gives a clear, clean scent over time. It is an oil which blends easily with others or can be used alone. Bergamot oil is extracted from the Bergamot Orange tree and has a fresh, fruity fragrance often used as a perfume material both in its natural form and synthetic substitute. It appears in about 40% of all women's perfumes. This particular splash is cleansing and refreshing and can be used as a base for creating many other custom fragrances.

Ingredients:

2 CUPS DISTILLED WATER

3 TABLESPOONS VODKA

15 DROPS SWEET ORANGE ESSENTIAL OIL

10 DROPS ESSENTIAL OIL OF BERGAMOT

ZEST FROM HALF A LEMON

- *Fill a sterilized jar with the zest.*

- *Pour water and vodka over zest and stir with a glass rod or stainless steel spoon.*

- *Add essential oils, seal with an airtight lid and set in a cool, dark place for one week, stirring every few days. Strain liquid through cheese cloth or a paper filter. Discard lemon zest.*

- *Stored in an amber glass bottle, Sweet Orange Splash can be kept for up to one year.*

LOUIS XV (18TH CENTURY) GAVE ORANGE BLOSSOM
WATER TO ALL THE LADIES OF THE COURT AT
VERSAILLES ON NEW YEAR'S DAY.

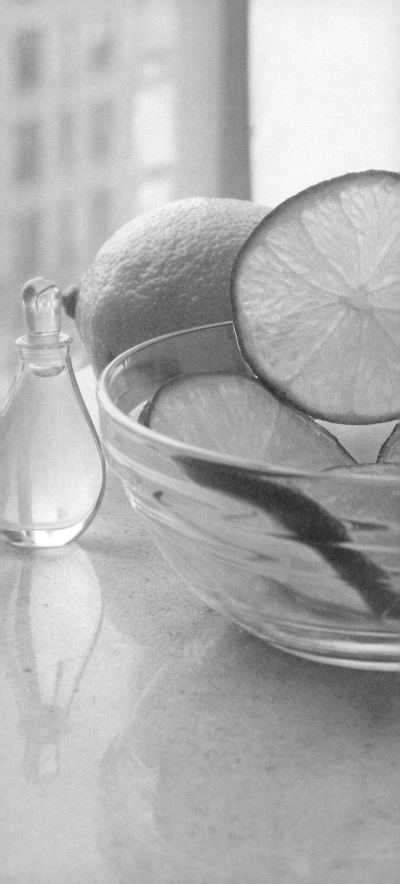

Lemon Lime Cologne

PROFILE
Fragrance Family: Citrus
Single Note: Citrus

T he highest quality lemon oil is extracted from the Yuzu Lemon tree of Japan, through a process of cold expression of the rind. With an unusually delicate fragrance that gives top notes a fresh sparkle and tangy scent, it is a common ingredient in eau de cologne. Coupled with lime oil, this delightfully refreshing cologne is perfect for summer evenings or for an imaginary walk in a citrus grove.

Ingredients:
1/2 CUP VODKA
1/2 CUP SWEET ORANGE SPLASH
(SEE RECIPE PAGE 143)
8 DROPS LEMON ESSENTIAL OIL
6 DROPS LIME ESSENTIAL OIL
ZEST FROM 1 LIME

- Prepare Sweet Orange Splash as indicated in recipe on page 143.

- In a large sterilized glass jar, mix vodka, lemon essential oil, lime essential oil, lime zest, and Sweet Orange Splash and stir with a glass rod or stainless steel spoon.

- Seal with an airtight lid and set aside in a cool, dark place for one week, stirring every two days.

- Strain through cheese cloth or a paper filter to remove zest.

- Store in an amber glass bottle and use within one year.

THE GREEK PHILOSOPHER PLATO CONSIDERED
PERFUMES TO BE IMMORAL AND THOUGHT THEY SHOULD
BE RESERVED UNIQUELY FOR PROSTITUTES.

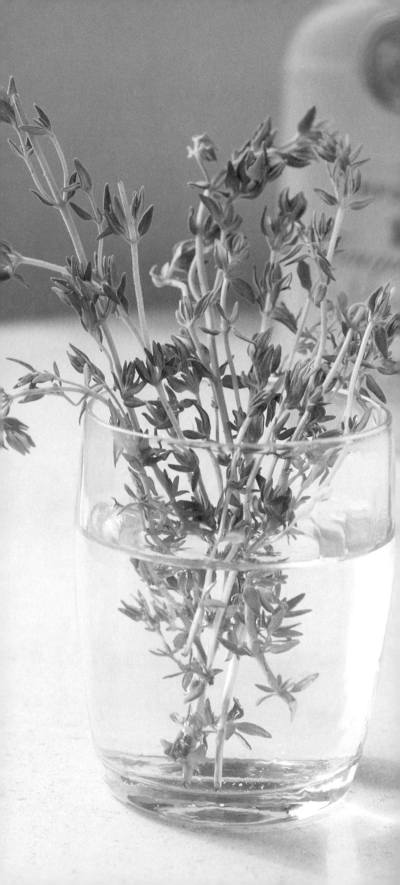

Clary Sage & Thyme Cologne

PROFILE

Fragrance Family: Chypre
Single Note: Cyprus

Clary sage oil, extracted from the Clary plant, is used in many perfumes and eau de colognes as an equilibrating agent in that it tones down and mellows out scents. It has been described as having a slightly nutty aroma with a note similar to musk, lavender and neroli. Thyme, which gets its name from the Greek "thymos" meaning "to perfume," has a rich, slightly sweet aroma that produces an herbal, green note in perfumery. White thyme oil, a refined version of the cruder red thyme oil distillate, is a common ingredient in the perfume industry. Clary Sage & Thyme Cologne provides comforting warmth on soggy, rainy days.

Ingredients:

1/2 CUP VODKA
10 DROPS CLARY SAGE ESSENTIAL OIL
5 DROPS THYME ESSENTIAL OIL

- *In a small sterilized glass jar, blend vodka with both essential oils and stir with a glass rod.*

- *Decant into a small amber glass bottle with a top or stopper and store in a cool place.*

- *Best when used within one year.*

DURING THE FIRST HALF OF THE 16TH CENTURY, THE PERFUME INDUSTRY WENT THROUGH A SERIOUS DECLINE. THE REFORMATION AND PURITANISM DECRIED ANYTHING THAT SMACKED OF AMUSEMENT OR PLEASURE: THEATER, FINE CLOTHES, FRAGRANCES, EXTRAVAGANT FOOD AND SPICES.

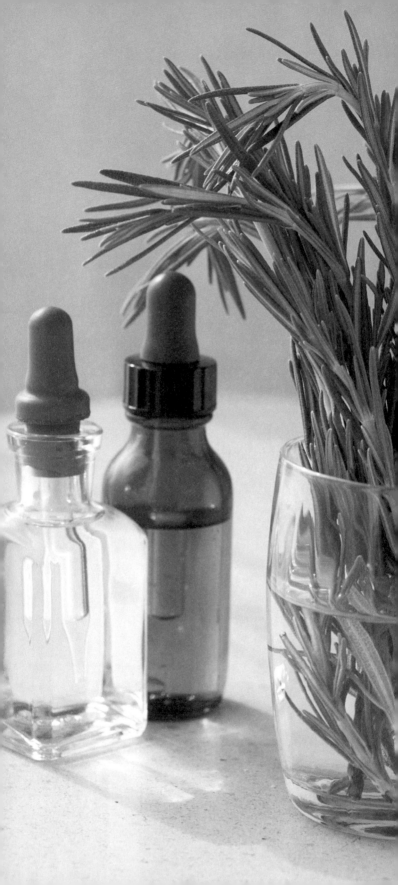

Oakmoss Perfume Blend

PROFILE

Fragrance Family: Chypre

Top Note: Citrus

Middle Note: Chypre

Base Note: Woody

O akmoss is a resin extracted from lichens found on various trees, particularly on oak trees. Oakmoss makes an excellent fixative and blends well with many oils, particularly lavender, jasmine, orange blossom and bergamot. It provides an earthy undertone to many perfumes on today's market. Rosemary, a principal ingredient in Hungary water which was created in 1370 for the Queen of Hungary, provides a fresh, clean scent that blends beautifully with the fruity, citrus fragrance of bergamot.

Ingredients:

1 TABLESPOON VODKA

10 DROPS OAKMOSS ESSENTIAL OIL

4 DROPS BERGAMOT ESSENTIAL OIL

4 DROPS ROSEMARY ESSENTIAL OIL

- *Blend ingredients in a small sterilized glass jar and stir with a glass rod.*

- *Decant into a small amber bottle with a top or stopper and store in a cool, dark place.*

- *Use within eight months.*

HUNGARY WATER, NAMED AFTER QUEEN ELIZABETH OF HUNGARY, WAS BASED ON OIL OF ROSEMARY AND LATER SOFTENED BY LAVENDER OIL.

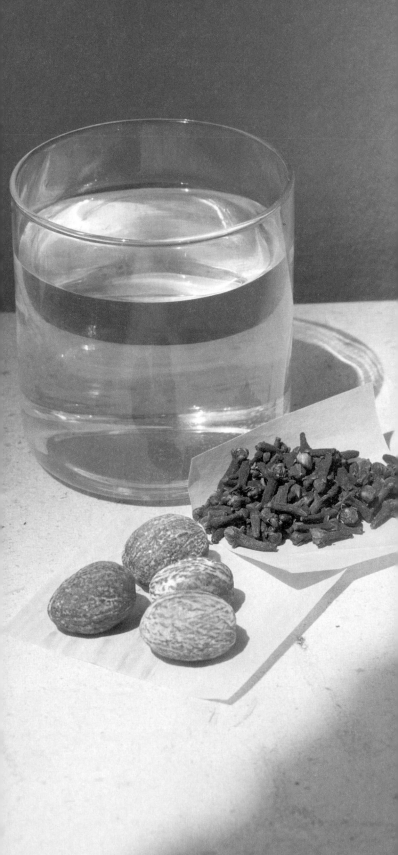

Spice Splash

PROFILE
Fragrance Family: Spicy
Single Note: Spicy/Woody

Nutmeg oil is distilled from the seeds of the nutmeg tree and is frequently used in the perfume industry to impart a musky note to fragrances, which balances out well with the sweetness of vanilla. The clove, the dried flower bud of the Clove tree, was one of the first ingredients used by the early Arab perfume makers, and is a key ingredient in many floral fragrances. Its essence provides the splash with subtle spicy undertones.

Ingredients:

1 CUP DISTILLED WATER

2 TABLESPOONS VODKA

5 DROPS NUTMEG ESSENTIAL OIL

5 DROPS VANILLA FRAGRANCE OIL

4 WHOLE CLOVES

- *In a sterilized jar with an airtight lid, blend water, vodka and whole cloves, and store in a cool, dark place for one week.*

- *Remove cloves and add nutmeg and vanilla oils.*

- *Decant in a small amber bottle with a top or stopper and store in a cool, dark place.*

- *Best when used within eight to ten months.*

LOUIS XIV HAD HIS PERFUMER,
MONSIEUR MARTIAL, CREATE A SPECIAL
PERFUME FOR HIM EVERY DAY.

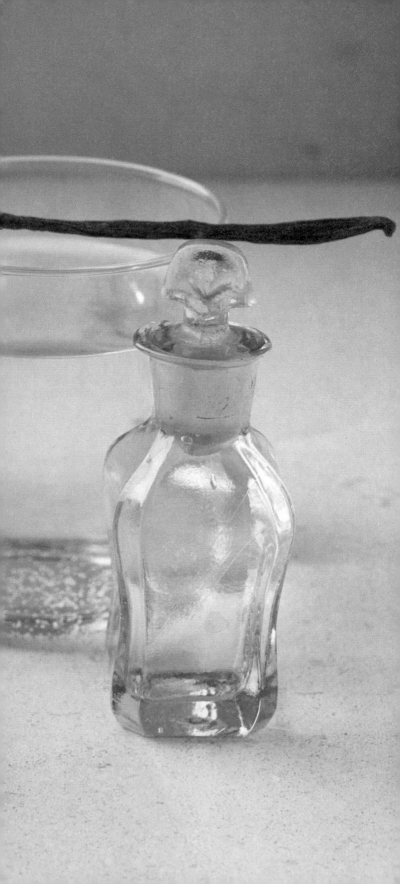

Vanilla Bean Water

PROFILE
Fragrance Family: Amber / Oriental
Top Note: Fruity / Spicy
Middle Note: Oriental

The vanilla bean was first discovered in Mexico by Cortés in the early 16th century. It owes its popularity in today's perfume industry to Francois Coty, recognized as one of the great perfumers of modern times. Coty was the first to use vanilla as a key fragrance ingredient in "L'Aimant," a fragrance he created in the late 1920s. Sandalwood is one of the oldest known perfumery materials, and was traditionally used in religious Chinese and Indian ceremonies, evidence of which dates as far back as the year 500 BC. Today, the tree is still protected and government-controlled in India, and it is used for its excellent fixative properties. Sandalwood oil has a woody, honey-like balsamic note, which retains its odor for a long time. The water's fragrance is warm, sensuous and long-lasting, yet not over powering.

Ingredients:

1 CUP DISTILLED WATER

2 TABLESPOONS VODKA

2 WHOLE VANILLA BEANS

5 DROPS SANDALWOOD ESSENTIAL OIL

- In a sterilized glass jar, blend water, vodka and vanilla bean. Seal with an airtight lid and allow to steep for one week.

- Remove vanilla bean and add sandalwood essential oil.

- Decant in an amber bottle with an airtight lid or stopper. Store in a cool, dark place and use within eight months.

❋

BEFORE GOING TO BATTLE, NAPOLEON TRADITIONALLY DRENCHED HIMSELF WITH COLOGNE. HE BELIEVED THAT THIS WAS NECESSARY TO MAINTAIN HIS PROWESS ON THE BATTLEFIELD.

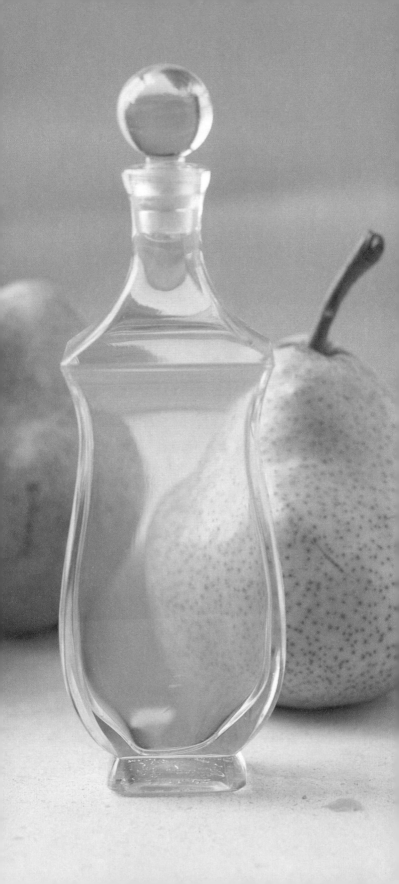

Pear Nectar Perfume

PROFILE
Fragrance Family: Floral / Oriental
Top Note: Citrus
Middle Note: Fruity
Base Note: Resinous

The combination of pear and neroli is truly mouth watering. Neroli oil, steam-distilled from the bitter orange tree, is light and citrusy sweet. Ann Maria Orsini, the Princess of Nerola, was notorious for scenting her baths and gloves with this delicate fragrance. The oil thus became very popular among the Italian aristocracy in the late 17th century and remains a common ingredient in today's perfumes and colognes. Frankincense (also known as olibanum) is a gum resin from the Boswellia trees of southern Saudi Arabia, Yemen and Africa. It has a deeply balsamic, fresh, resinous aroma, with an occasional green apple-like note. The resin is often used as a fixative in the perfume industry, specifically in the creation of fragrances with strong oriental notes. This long lasting scent is also said to have aphrodisiac powers, so wear it with caution.

Ingredients:
1 TABLESPOON VODKA
8 DROPS PEAR FRAGRANCE OIL
4 DROPS NEROLI ESSENTIAL OIL
4 DROPS FRANKINCENSE ESSENTIAL OIL

- *In a sterilized glass jar, blend vodka, fragrance and essential oils and stir gently with a glass rod or stainless steel spoon.*

- *Decant in an amber bottle with a top or lid and store in a cool, dark place. Use within eight months to one year.*

IN PERFUMERY, AN INDIVIDUAL WHO PLAYS WITH AND COMBINES NOTES TO CREATE A SCENT IS KNOWN AS A "NOSE". A "NOSE" IS ABLE TO RECOGNIZE AND MIX MORE THAN 2000 DIFFERENT SCENTS

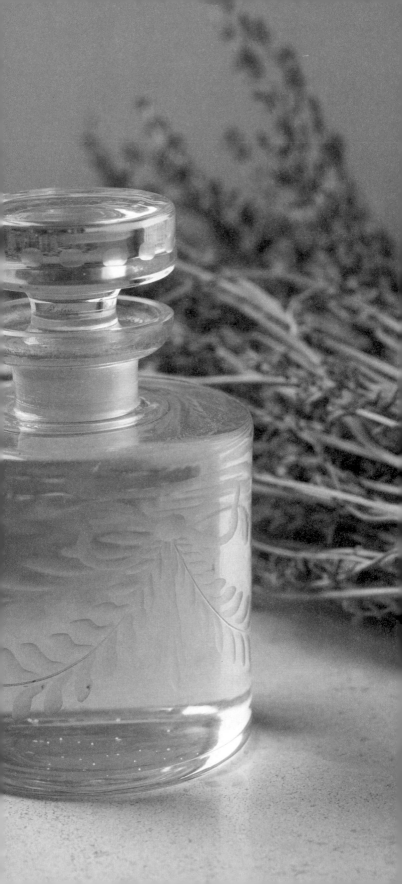

Provence Perfume Oil

PROFILE
Fragrance Family: Floral
Top Note: Floral
Middle Note: Floral
Base Note: Floral

Perfume oil does not have as long a shelf life as fragrances that are made with alcohol, but certain individuals prefer its unctuous consistency. Perfume oil is also notorious for having a longer staying power than most alcohol-based fragrances. Sweet almond or jojoba oil is an ideal base for carrying scents in perfume oils. However as their shelf life tends to be shorter than other oils, it is best to use perfume oils within the first six months.

The scent of lavender is very distinct—some say it's addictive. It has been a popular perfume material since ancient Greek and Roman times. Lavender oil is extracted from the flowering tips of the shrub by steam distillation. It takes about 3,600 plants of English Lavender (which has the finest aroma of the various types of lavender) or one acre of plants to produce 15 pounds of oil. Most of the lavender oil produced today comes from Provence, a region in the South of France. If you have ever walked through or driven by a purple field of lavender, this particular perfume oil will take you back in no time.

Ingredients:
1 TEASPOON SWEET ALMOND OIL
15 DROPS LAVENDER ESSENTIAL OIL
10 DROPS SANDALWOOD ESSENTIAL OIL

- *Blend ingredients in a sterilized glass jar and decant into an amber bottle with an airtight lid or stopper.*

- *Store in a cool, dark place and use within six months.*

THE HUMAN NOSE CAN DETECT (BUT NOT NECESSARILY RECOGNIZE) OVER 10,000 DIFFERENT ODORS.

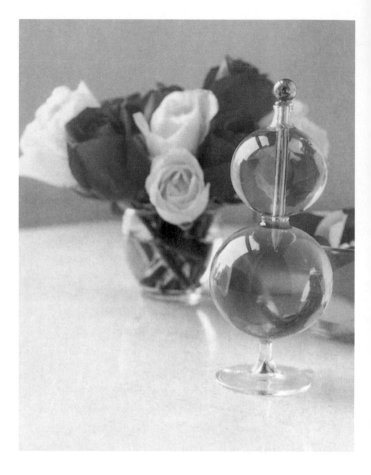

- Ancient Egyptians created kyphi, a perfumed substance in the shape of a cone which was placed on a person's head and gradually melted at body temperature and perfuming the face and neck.

- The Greeks were the first to introduce the use of perfume for personal rather than religious reasons.

- In addition to using fragrances on their clothing and linens, the Romans perfumed the sails of their ships.

- Egyptian men and women put perfumed lotions and oils in their hair.

- Assyrians perfumed their beards.

- In 1573 the Earl of Oxford presented Queen Elizabeth with a pair of scented gloves, thereby shepherding into existence the fragrance industry in England.

- During the reign of King George III, perfume was regarded as so powerfully seductive that an act was published stating: "All women that shall seduce or betray into matrimony any of His Majesty's subjects by scents, paints, cosmetic washes… shall incur the penalty of the law in force against witchcraft… and the marriage, upon conviction, shall stand null and void."

- Catherine de Medici created a fashion for perfumed gloves in 16th century France and until the reign of Louis XIV (who, by the way, was known as the "Sweet Smelling Monarch") perfume sales were a branch of the glove manufacturer's industry.

- In 18th century France, scented woodwork decorated the walls of boudoirs.

- Before going to battle, Napoleon traditionally drenched himself with a full bottle of cologne and tucked a flask of it in his boot. He believed that this was necessary to maintain his prowess on the battlefield.

- Cologne bottles were first made in about 1830 and toilet-water bottles in the 1880's.

- Francois Coty was one of the first to package perfume in crystal bottles: Ambre Antique (a 1905 Coty perfume) appears in a Lalique bottle.

- In the 1920s, Coco Chanel took women out of their stiff corsets and put them into comfortable, easy-to-wear clothes with clean, simple lines. Chanel's look characterized the spirit of her fragrances as well: fresh, new and innovative. Chanel N° 5 was released in 1921.

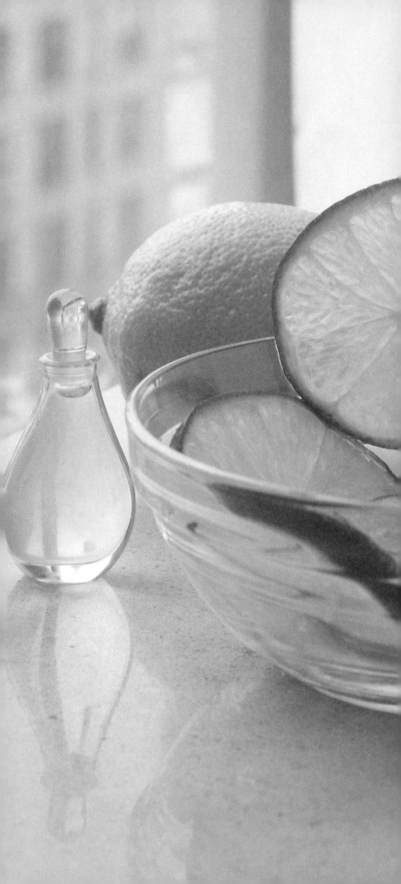

- The individual who plays with and combines notes to create a scent is known as a "nose." A professional "nose" can recognize and mix more than 2,000 different scents.

- An average fragrance has 60 to 100 ingredients-more complex fragrances can have 300.

- There are only about 400 perfumers in the world; more than half work in the U.S.

- Orris, which comes from the rhizome of an iris, is the most expensive natural material at $40,000 a pound.

- There are approximately 20 different rose notes.

- Scent is composed of evaporating molecules which are converted by the human nose into smell.

- On an average day, the average human nose comes in contact with and recognizes over 40 scents (shampoos, soaps, lotions, deodorants, etc.)

- Scientists have found that olfactory neurons in the olfactory epithelium only survive for about 60 days. But as olfactory neurons die, a new layer of olfactory neurons is generated to maintain a steady supply.

- Each individual has her/his own smell fingerprint, that is determined by skin type, hair color, diet, stress, etc.

- Oily skin holds fragrances longer than dry skin.

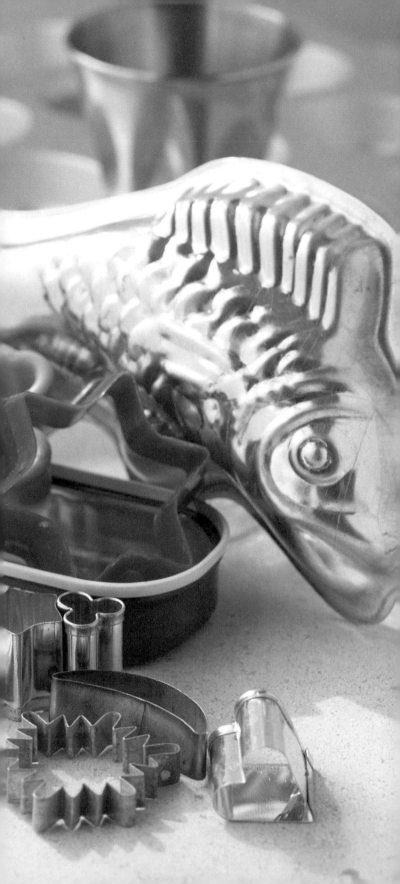

Essentials

ESSENTIAL OILS

·

SAPONIFICATION CHART

·

GLOSSARY

·

RESOURCES, SUPPLIERS AND MANUFACTURERS

·

BIBLIOGRAPHY

·

CONVERSION TABLE

·

YOUR OWN CUSTOM BLENDS

Essential oils are natural substances that are extracted from grasses, flowers, herbs, shrubs, trees, resins and spices, usually through a process called steam distillation. Their aromatic effect, when used to scent soaps, splashes and perfumes can soothe, relax, rejuvenate, heal, energize or relieve pain, thereby affecting the body's physical, psychological and emotional levels.

SAFETY TIPS

- Essential oils should be stored in amber glass bottles away from direct sunlight and in a cool place. Never store an essential oil in a plastic bottle.
- If you store oils in the refrigerator, place the bottles in air-tight containers so that the aroma does not permeate food.
- Certain oils may solidify in cold temperatures due to their high wax content. If this occurs, place the oil bottle in a bowl of hot water to liquefy before use.
- Most essential oils have a shelf life of two years, with the exception of pine and citrus oils which lose some of their potency after 6 months.
- The color of certain oils may change with time; this does not affect the potency of the oil.
- Avoid using essential oils around the eye area.
- Never apply an essential oil directly to the skin; dilute it first (see below for dilution rates).
- Never use internally unless under the supervision and care of a specialist.
- Essential oils are not recommended for babies and small children and should always be stored out of the reach of children.

The following is a chart of the most essential of the essential oils and a brief description of their properties. Oils can be purchased at health food stores or by mail order.

NAME / LATIN NAME	PROPERTIES & SAFETY PRECAUTIONS
Ajowan *Trachyspermum copticum*	improves circulation, alleviates muscle pain • *use sparingly on sensitive skin*
Angelica *Angelica archangelica*	strengthening, restorative, anchoring • *avoid use in sun*
Aniseed *Pimpinella anisum*	aids in cramping, indigestion or digestive problems • *do not use if pregnant*
Armoise *Artimisia alba*	muscle relaxant, emollient • *do not use if pregnant*
Basil *Ocimum basilicum*	soothing agent, muscle relaxant, toning • *use sparingly*
Bay *Pimenta racemosa*	stimulating, energizing • *can cause skin irritation*
Bergamot *Citrus bergamia*	skin conditioner, soothing agent, antiseptic • *phototoxic*
Birch Tar *Betula lenta*	muscle relaxant, soothing agent • *do not use if pregnant*
Black Currant Seed *Ribes nigrum*	relieves PMS, high source of vitamin C
Black Pepper *Piper nigrum*	muscle relaxant
Cabreuva *Myocarpus fastigiatus*	calming, increases alertness
Cajeput *Melaleuca cajuputi*	stimulating, mood improving, antiseptic
Camphor *Cinnamon camphor*	soothing agent, conditioner, muscle relaxant • *do not use if pregnant or epileptic*
Cananga *Cananga odorata*	skin conditioner, deodorant
Caraway *Carum carvi*	muscle relaxant • *slight dermal toxicity*
Cardamom *Elettaria cardamomum*	muscle relaxant, skin conditioner, soothing agent
Carrot Seed *Daucus carota*	muscle relaxant, soothing agent, skin conditioner
Cedarwood Virginia *Juniperis virginiana*	antiseptic, skin conditioner, deodorant, soothing agent
Celery Seed *Apium graveolens*	toner
Chamomile Moroc *Anthemis mixta*	muscle relaxant, skin conditioner
Chamomile Roman *Anthemis noblis*	muscle relaxant, skin conditioner
Cinnamon Bark *Cinnamomum zeylanicum*	skin conditioner, anti-inflammatory agent • *can cause skin irritation*
Citronella *Cymbopogon nardus*	skin conditioner, insect repellent
Clary Sage *Salvia sclarea*	skin conditioner, astringent, soothing agent, muscle relaxant • *do not use if pregnant; do not drink alcohol or drive*
Clove Bud *Syzgium aromaticum*	muscle relaxant, soothing agent • *can cause skin irritation*

NAME / LATIN NAME	PROPERTIES & SAFETY PRECAUTIONS
Copaiba Balsam *Copaifera officinalis*	increases circulation, reduces stress
Coriander *Corriandrum sativum*	muscle relaxant, soothing agent • *use sparingly*
Costus Root *Sassuriea costus*	calming
Cumin *Cuminum cyminum*	stimulating • *can cause skin irritation*
Cypress *Cupressus sempervirens*	antiseptic, astringent, soothing agent, skin conditioner • *flammable*
Cypriol *Cyperus scariosus*	aids digestion
Eucalyptus *Eucalyptus globulus*	antiseptic, soothing agent, skin conditioner, insect repellent
Evening Primrose *Centhera biennis*	good for dry skin and eczema
Fennel (sweet) *Foeniculum vulgare dulce*	muscle relaxant, soothing agent, antiseptic • *use sparingly*
Frankincense *Boswellia carteri*	skin conditioner, soothing agent
Galbanum *Ferula galbaniflua*	skin conditioner, muscle relaxant
Geranium *Pelargonium graveolen*	skin refresher, astringent
Ginger *Zingiber officinale*	astringent
Grapefruit *Citrus paradisi*	soothing agent, astringent, skin conditioner
Hyssop *Hyssopus officinalis*	soothing agent, skin conditioner • *do not use when pregnant, if suffering from* *epilepsy or high blood pressure*
Jasmine Absolute *Jasminum officinale*	emollient, soothing agent, antiseptic
Juniper *Juniperus communis*	skin detoxifier, astringent, soothing agent • *flammable*
Labdanum *Cistus ladanifer*	skin conditioner
Lavandin *Lavandula hybrida*	soothing agent, muscle relaxant, skin conditioner, astringent
Lavender *Lavandula officinalis*	muscle relaxant, skin conditioner, soothing agent, astringent
Lemon *Citrus limonum*	soothing agent, antiseptic
Lemongrass *Cymbopogon flexuosus*	skin conditioner, soothing agent, muscle relaxant, antiseptic • *can cause skin irritation*
Lime *Citrus aurantifolia*	soothing agent, skin conditioner, astringent
Mandarin *Citrus reticulata*	soothing agent, astringent, skin conditioner
Manuka *Leptospermum*	relieves aches and pains, healing to the skin
Marjoram *Origanum marjorana*	antiseptic, calming
Mimosa *Acacia dealbata*	muscle relaxant, skin conditioner, soothing agent
Myrrh *Commiphora myrrha*	anti-inflammatory agent, emollient, antiseptic • *use in moderation if pregnant*

NAME / LATIN NAME	PROPERTIES & SAFETY PRECAUTIONS
Myrtle *Myrtus communis*	soothing agent, astringent, skin conditioner, muscle relaxant
Neroli *Citrus aurantium*	antiseptic, emollient
Nutmeg Myristica fragrans *Niaouli elaleuca viridiflora*	antiseptic, soothes irritated skin, muscle relaxant • **use sparingly**
Orange *Citrus sinensis*	astringent, soothing agent, skin conditioner
Origanum *Origanum vulgare*	increases energy • **can cause skin irritation**
Palmarosa *Cymbopogon martini*	skin conditioner, soothing agent, emollient, muscle relaxant
Patchouli *Pogostemon cablin*	anti-inflammatory agent, antiseptic, astringent
Peppermint *Mentha arvensis*	emollient, antiseptic, muscle relaxant • **can cause skin irritation**
Petitgrain *Petitgrain bigarade*	relieves anxiety and stress
Pine *Pinus sylvestris*	antiseptic • **can cause skin irritation**
Rose Absolute *Rosa damascena*	skin conditioner
Rose Otto *Rosa*	astringent
Rosemary *Rosmarinus officinalis*	antiseptic, muscle relaxant, soothing agent, skin conditioner • **do not take if pregnant or have high blood pressure**
Rosewood *Aniba rosaeodora*	muscle relaxant
Sage *Dalmatian Salvia officinalis*	soothing agent • **do not use if pregnant or suffering from epilepsy**
Sandalwood *(Mysore) Sandalum album*	antiseptic, emollient, soothing agent, astringent, skin conditioner
Spearmint *Mentha spicata*	emollient, astringent, soothing agent, muscle relaxant • **use sparingly**
Tarragon *Artimisia dracunculus*	astringent
Tea Tree *Melaleuca alternifolia*	antiseptic • **may cause irritation to sensitive skin**
Thyme *Thymus vulgaris*	antiseptic, toner • **can cause skin irritation**
Vanilla *Vanilla planifolia*	emollient
Vetiver *Vetiveria zizanioides*	emollient, reduces blood pressure
Violet Leaves *Viola*	soothing agent, skin conditioner
Yarrow *Achillea millefolium*	reduces scarring
Ylang-Ylang *Cananga odorata*	reduces stress and tension
Zanthoxylum *Zanthoxylum alatum*	reduces stress and tension

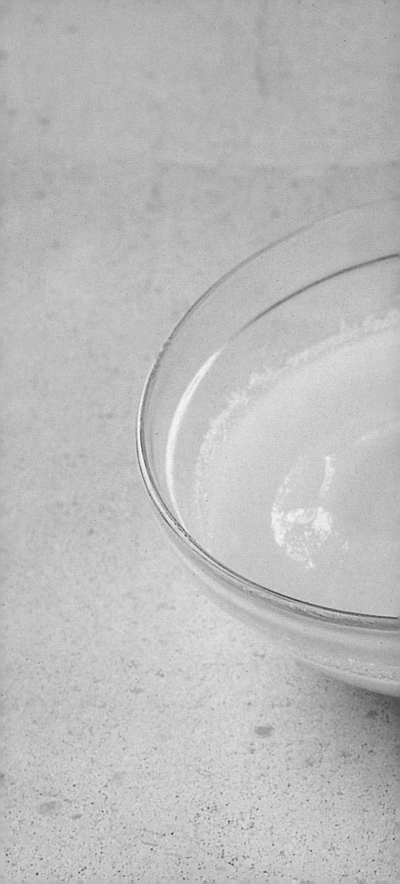

Saponification Chart

The saponification value (SAP value) of a particular oil or fat is the amount of potassium hydroxide (caustic potash) in milligrams needed to saponify one gram of that oil or fat. The metric system is used because these figures are based on the molecular weight of specific compounds, and molecular weight is universally measured in milligrams.

In order to obtain the amount of sodium hydroxide (lye or caustic soda) required to saponify that oil or fat, take the amount of potassium hydroxide that would be needed then multiply it by 0.71. (In case you're wondering, the number 0.71 was obtained by a multiple step calculation involving molecular weights of various compounds. We've opted to spare you a chemistry class by skipping the details.) Don't worry; we've made it easy.

Each oil or fat has a different SAP value; therefore it takes different amounts of potassium hydroxide (and hence sodium hydroxide) to saponify different fats and oils.

The SAP value of coconut oil for example is 268.0. This means that it takes 268.0 milligrams of potassium hydroxide to saponify 1,000 milligrams (or 1 gram) of coconut oil. To get the amount of lye needed, you then multiply 268.0 by 0.71 for a total of 191.2 milligrams.

FAT OR OIL per 1,000 MG or 1G	SAP VALUE amount of potassium hydroxide needed in MG	amount of lye or sodium hydroxide needed in MG
Almond Oil	192.5	137.2
Apricot Kernel Oil	190.0	135.5
Avocado Oil	187.5	133.7
Beef Tallow	197.0	140.5
Calendula Oil	190.0	137.5
Castor Oil	180.3	128.5
Cocoa Butter	193.8	138.2
Coconut Oil	268.0	191.2
Corn Oil	192.0	129.8
Evening Primrose Oil	191.0	136.2
Hazelnut Oil	195.0	139.0
Jojoba Oil	97.5	69.5
Lard	194.6	138.7
Macadamia Nut Oil	195.0	139.0
Olive Oil	189.7	135.2
Palm Kernel Oil	219.9	156.8
Palm Oil	199.1	141.9
Peanut Oil	192.1	136.9
Safflower Oil	192.0	136.9
Sesame Oil	187.9	133.9
Shea Butter	180.0	128.3
Soybean Oil	190.6	135.9
Sunflower Seed Oil	188.7	134.5
Sweet Almond Oil	192.5	137.2
Wheat Germ Oil	185.0	131.9

Crisco   *123.29* (handwritten)

WAX		
Beeswax	88.0	62.7
Lanolin	82.0	58.5
Lecithin	110.0	78.4

THE BASICS

- When working with a combination of oils, you need to determine the SAP value for the mixture. For example, suppose you are combining 7 grams of coconut oil with 3 grams of shea butter, for a total of 10 grams (or 1000 milligrams) of oils.

- To calculate the combined SAP value, you have to figure in the SAP value of each oil and the percentage each oil contributes to the total weight of the fats/oils.

- So for the 7 grams of coconut oil and the 3 grams of shea butter, it would be: 0.7 multiplied by 268.0 plus 0.3 multiplied by 180.0 for a total of 241.6 milligrams. The combined SAP value of the fats/oils is 241.6.

- Multiply the total weight of the fats/oils by the combined SAP value to get the total mount of potassium hydroxide needed:

- 10 grams multiplied by 0.2416 grams for a total of 2.41 grams of potassium hydroxide needed

- For the amount of sodium hydroxide/lye needed, multiply 2.41 by 0.71:

- 2.41 multiplied by 0.71 for a total of 1.71 grams of sodium hydroxide needed for an oil mixture in which there are 7 grams of coconut oil and 3 grams of shea butter

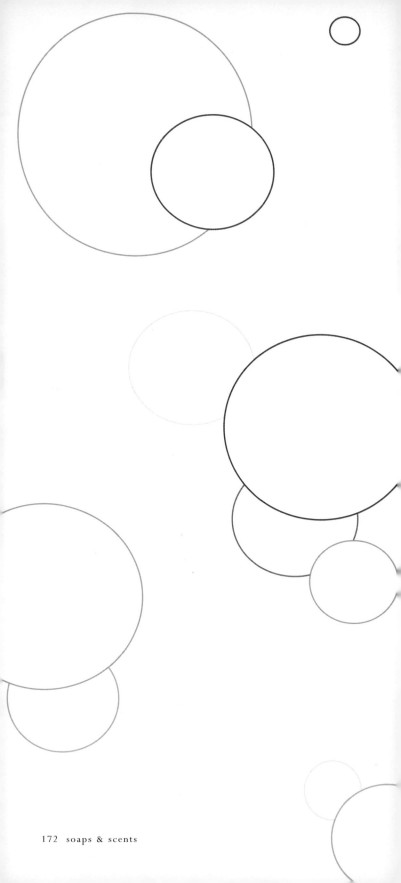

GLOSSARY OF TERMS AND TECHNIQUES

*=Words, terms and expressions commonly
used in the fragrance industry

•=Words, terms and expressions commonly
used in the soap industry

* **Abir** an aromatic powder of Hindu origin,
composed primarily of clove, sandalwood,
and cardamom, which is frequently used
to perfume oriental products.

• **Absolute** a highly concentrated extract of
perfumery material (derived from a flower,
piece of bark, or leaf, for example), which
is free from waxes and other by-products.
It has on average undergone at least two
extraction processes.

• **Acid Value** the amount of potassium
hydroxide needed to neutralize the fatty
acid in one gram of fatty material.

* **Accord** a complex blend of three or four
scents (or notes) which, individually, carry
a distinctive identity and aroma but when
blended together, lose their individuality to
create an entirely new scent with a char-
acteristic and aromatic identity of its own.

* **Alcohol** denatured ethyl alcohol is added
to perfumery material or perfume oil to
modify its intensity. The less a material is
diluted with alcohol, the more powerful the
odor impression. The most concentrated
fragrances (highest percentage of perfume
oil to alcohol) to the least concentrated
fragrances (lowest percentage of perfume
oil to alcohol) are as follows:

Extract of perfume
96 proof alcohol combined with oil to a
concentration greater than 22 percent
perfume oil

Eau de toilette
80 to 90 proof alcohol to a concentration
of 8 to 15 percent perfume oil

Eau de cologne
50 to 75 proof alcohol to a concentration
of up to 5 percent perfume oil

* **Aldehyde** a synthetically or naturally
derived organic chemical used
primarily in the manufacture of synthetic
fragrances. Aldehyde-based fragrances
tend to leave rich and mysterious
odorous impressions or top notes.
In 1921, Coco Chanel's Nº 5 was the
first perfume to successfully perfect
the use of aldehydes in its manufacture.

• **Alkali** a substance with a pH higher than
7. Sodium hydroxide is an alkali that is
used to neutralize an acid to make soap.

* **Amber** resin obtained from fir trees wand
gives fragrances a warm note; a fragrance
family that is characterized by warm,
woody, sweet, exotic scents.

* **Ambergris** a light, almost odorless and
slightly greasy substance formed in the
intestines of sperm whales. This substance was commonly used as a fixing
agent in perfumes to impart a rich, smoky,
velvet and musk-like fragrance. In modern
perfumery, ambergrisóas well as other ani-
mal-derived substances such as musk,
castor or civet – is used sparingly.
Instead, these warm animal notes are
mimicked through the use of certain
plants and chemicals.

* **Animalic** a term used to describe a fragrance that is literally animal in
origin such as musk, castor, civet, or
ambergris.

* **Anosmia** the medical term for the loss of
the sense of smell.

* **Apocrine** a type of sweat gland in
the human body that determines an
individual's body odor and affects the way
a fragrance smells on different individuals.

* **Attar, attar,** or **otto** comes from the
Persian word Atr jul which means "fat of a
flower." It is the essential oil derived from
a flower by distillation. Usually used in
context with rose essential oils.

* **Balance** the result of blending
fragrance components into a well-blended
and harmonious sensory impression.

* **Balsam** a resin extracted from trees and
shrubs used in perfumery primarily as a
fixative.

• **Base** the alkali (usually sodium hydroxide
or lye) used to react with the fats or oils to
make soap.

* **Base notes** these notes, also called low
notes or back notes, define a fragrance's
tenacity and staying power. The ingredients in these notes, which are the longest
lasting, are generally referred to as fixatives.

^ **Baudruchage** a method used by certain
perfumers to seal bottles. The neck and
stopper if the bottle are covered and

joined by a thin membrane (traditionally pig intestine) then a thin thread is knotted around the membrane and serves as a seal.
* **Blotter Strip** *see mouillette*

• **Chlorophyll** found in plants, a substance often used as a soap coloring. It also provides the soap with antiseptic properties.

* **Chypre** a fragrance family mostly based on woody notes such as clary sage, oakmoss, and patchouli

* **Citrus** a term used to describe a type of note, specifically that of oranges, lemons, limes, mandarins, neroli and bergamot.

• **Cold process** a basic soap making process, which involves the reaction of fats/oils with lye to make soap.

* **Cold steeping** a method of oil extraction that later became known as enfleurage. See enfleurage

* **Cologne** a light fragrance with low concentrations of perfume oils in an alcohol base.

* **Concrete** a waxy substance obtained by the extraction of essential oils through the use of volatile solvents. Concretes can undergo further distillation and purification, producing absolutes. See absolute

• **Curing** an aging process (usually 4 to 8 weeks) after the soap has been poured into the moulds. During the curing stage, saponification continues (the lye is still active) rendering a mild bar.

* **Depth** used to describe the richness and fullness of a fragrance.

* **Dry down** the final phase of a fragrance's life (after application) in which the base notes can be properly evaluated.

* **Dry note** a note that connotes a woodsy or mossy fragrance.

* **Eau de Toilette** a perfume preparation that has a perfume oil concentration of 4-8 percent.

• **Emollient** a substance that holds in the skin's moisture and prevents water loss.

* **Enfleurage** a method of extracting essential oils or absolutes from plants or flowers by saturating them in animal fat. Once the fat is saturated, it is then mixed with alcohol, heated and cooled. The mixture is then filtered to remove all fats and plant or flower residue, the alcohol is evaporated, leaving the essential oil.

•* **Essential oils** concentrated essences derived from plants, bark, roots, seeds, stems, flowers, fruits and leaves through a method of extraction, usually steam distillation.

•* **Expression** a cold pressing method used to extract essential oils from fruits, usually citrus. The rinds are pressed between rollers or hydraulic presses to remove the oils from them.

* **Extraction** the process in which ingredients such as flowers, plants, seeds, etc. are added to a volatile solvent and heated at low temperatures which releases the ingredient's oils into the solvent. The solvent is evaporated, leaving the oil.

* **Extract** a concentrated form of plant materia.l

* **Extrait** the purest form of perfume with the highest concentration of fragrance oils in alcohol.

* **Factice** a dummy perfume bottle, sometimes oversized, filled with a tinted liquid to simulate a fragrance, and generally used for display purposes.

* **Fixative** a substance that prolongs the rate at which an odor evaporates. They are often derived from mosses, resins and aroma chemicals. Common fixatives include cedarwood chips, orange peel orris root, patchouli, storax oil, and clary sage. See also base note.

* **Flacon** a small perfume bottle with an airtight ornamental stopper.

* **Floral** a fragrance family that is characterized by scents derived from flowers; a term used to describe notes and fragrances that are derived from flowers.

•* **Fragrance oils** synthetic imitations of essential oils.

• **Glycerin** a by-product of the soap-making process, this substance is often re-added to soap because of its naturally emollient qualities. Soaps that have a great deal of glycerin in them are often transparent.

* **Green** a fragrance family characterized by fresh, herbal scents; a term used to describe fragrances that smell like freshly moved lawns and green plants in general.

* **Gum** a sticky substance that comes from parts of trees or shrubs, generally used as a bonding agent or fixative.
* **Heart** the core of a fragrance; that which defines its character.

* **Intensity** the strength or impact of a fragrance; unrelated to duration or quality.

* **Incense** a fragrant smoke produced by burning aromatic materials and substances.

* **Ionones** a chemical substance essential to violet perfumes and fragrances.

* **Limbic system** an area of the brain that receives messages from the olfactory nerves and interprets them. The limbic system is the seat of emotions, moods, and sex drive

* **Lye** also known as caustic soda or sodium hydroxide, a key element in the soapmaking process in that it forms the caustic alkali or base which reacts with fats and oils to produce soap. Lye is available commercially in pellets, sticks, or chips and should be handled with care as direct contact with skin will cause burning and irritation.

* **Maceration** an essential oil extraction method by which flowers are steeped in large vats of hot fats. The mixture is then washed in alcohol and the alcohol is evaporated, leaving the oil.

* **Middle note** the note – also called the heart, or body – of the fragrance that determines which family it belongs to. Middle notes take anywhere from 8 to 16 minutes after application to fully develop on the skin.

* **Modern** a fragrance family that refers to blends containing aldehydes which enhance the scents of other components in the fragrance. Modern fragrances have a rich top note, and an overall powdery appeal. Chanel No 5, created by Ernest Beaux, was the first perfume in which aldehydes were used in this manner.

* **Mouillette** a thin strip of absorbent filter paper used to evaluate a fragrance.

* **Note** term used to represent the varying stages of evaporation of essential oils. Basically, a note is the key to how a fragrance smells on the skin once it's applied and hours later. There are 3 categories of notes top notes, which are the most prominent scents when you first smell a perfume; middle notes, which surface once top notes have begun to fade away; and base notes which give the fragrance its endurance.

* **Oceanic** a fragrance family based on synthetic materials that are reminiscent of natural scents like freshly washed linen, ocean breeze or mountain air.

* **Olfactory** relating to the sense of smell.

* **Olfactory bulb** a pea-size region of the brain that receives sensory input or electrical messages from the olfactory neurons and sends them to other areas of the brain through the limbic system.

* **Olfactory cell** a neuron that senses odorant molecules.

* **Olfactory epithelium** a layer of receptor cells (*see vomeronasal organs*) which line the upper rear portion of the nose. These are the "smell sensors" which transmit the electrical message to the olfactory bulb. The olfactory epithelium contains more than 5 million olfactory neurons.

* **Olfactory recognition threshold** the lowest concentration of a vapor that can be detected and identified correctly.

* **Perfume concentration** refers to the percentage of essential oils contained in the perfume's composition.

* **Perfume dip sticks** see mouillette

* **pH** is a measure of the hydrogen ion concentration of a substance.
    - pH of 7 is balanced
    - pH between 1 and 7 is acidic
    - pH between 7 and 14 is basic or alkaline

* **Pheromone** chemical substance secreted by animals to produce a response by other animals of the same species.

* **Pomade** a perfumed ointment used on skin and hair. Perfumers use it to describe a substance made out of fat and the scent of flowers, a substance crucial to the enfleurage process.

* **Rendering** the process by which fat is cleaned and purified — the final product is tallow.

* **Resinoid** a resin which has been purified with alcohol to remove sticky materials.

• **Saponification** a complex chemical reaction in which a fatty acid reacts to a base to produce soap and glycerin.

• **Saponification value** (SAP) the SAP value of an oil is equivalent to the amount of potassium hydroxide needed to saponify one gram of that oil.

• **Separation** a term used to describe a trouble sign in the soap-making process in which the oils separate from the lye mixture.

• **Soap** the product that results from the reaction of a fatty acid (fats or oils) and a strong base (of which sodium hydroxide is the most common).

* **Solvents** volatile fluids that are used to extract essential oils from plants, flower, herbs, and other natural perfume materials.

* **Spicy** a fragrance family characterized by spicy scents nutmeg, cinnamon, cloves, cassia, etc.

* **Splash cologne** a toilet water containing between 1% and 3% of perfume concentrate.

* **Steam distillation** the most popular method used for extracting essential oils from flowers, plants, bark, seeds and fruit.

* **Strength** the intensity of a fragrance.

• **Superfatting** adding excess oils or fats to soap to make it rich and creamier. This process occurs after tracing but before pouring the soap mixture into molds. Avocado oil and cocoa butter are often used, separately, as superfatting agents.

* **Synthetic Fragrances** laboratory made imitations of natural perfumes, or fragrances that are fabricated in a lab and do not exist in nature.

• **Tallow** pure animal fat after impurities have been removed.

* **Tenacity** a fragrance or a note's ability to last. Also known as substantivity

• **Titer** the temperature at which fatty acids from a fat or oil solidify; i.e. solidification temperature. The higher a fat or oil's titer, the harder the soap.

* **Toilette water** *see eau de toilette*

* **Top note** the first impression of a fragrance right after it has been applied to the skin; of all three notes—top, middle and base—top notes are the most volatile and evaporate first.

* **Tracing** a term used in soapmaking that indicates when soap is ready to be poured into molds. When the water/lye solution and the fat first combine, the mixture is watery. As the fat and lye react with each other, the mixture starts to thicken and turns opaque. Tracing is complete when you can draw a line of soap in the mixture with a spoon or spatula, or when a design forms on the surface when you let the mixture drizzle off the spoon.

* **Undertones** the background subtlety of a fragrance

• **Unsaponifiables** oils, which do not participate in the soapmaking reaction and are left intact in the final bar of soap.

* **Volatile** a substance that is easily vaporized at low temperatures; a term that refers to the lifespan of a note a highly volatile note evaporates very quickly.

* **Vomeronasal organs** nerve cells in tiny cigar-shaped sacs located in the olfactory epithelium, just behind the nostril, in the nose's dividing wall. These organs contain receptor cells that pick up chemical signals and then transmit them through the limbic system to the olfactory bulb.

* **Woody** a term used to describe a fragrance that has a rich, deep aroma reminiscent of wood, but are not necessarily extracted from wood. Examples are sandalwood, musk, cedar, patchouli, vetiver or oak.

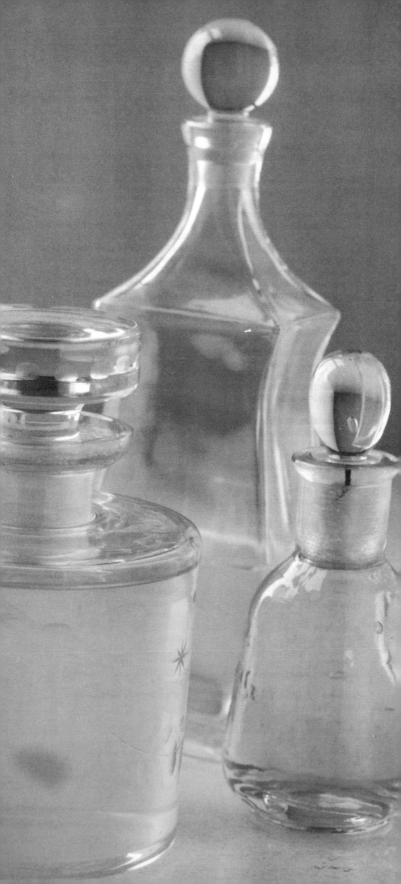

RESOURCES, SUPPLIERS AND ASSOCIATIONS

USEFUL WEBSITES

Soap:

Brookside Soap Making Supplies
www.halcyon.com/brookside/makesupp.htm

National Craft Association
www.craftassoc.com/ssoap.html

Sugar Plum Sundries
www.craftassoc.com/ssoap.html

Soap Crafters Company
www.soapcrafters.com

Creation Herbal Products
www.creationsoap@boone.net

Sweetcakes Soap Making Supplies
www.sweetcakes.com

Fine Handcrafted Soap by the Soap Factory
www.alcasoft.com/soapfact

Countryside Soap
www.countrysidesoap.com

Au Natural Handmade Soaps and Sundries
www.simplerway.com/au-naturale

Natural Way Soapworks
www.localaccess.com/NaturalWaySoap

Savon de Marseille
www.marseillesoap.com/index.htm

Greek Olive Warehouse Imports, Inc.
www.greekolivewarehouse.com/chiamp/soaps

Pourette
6910 Roosevelt Way NE
Seattle, WA 98115
(206) 525-4488
(general soap-making supplies)

Angel's Earth
1633 Scheffer Avenue
St. Paul, MN 55116
(612) 698-3636
(general soap-making supplies, oils)

Sunfeather Herbal Soap Company, Inc.
1551 State Highway 72
Potsdam, New York 13676
(general soap-making supplies, oils)

House of Crafts
62 Knighton Lane
Leicester LE2 8BG
01 16 283 8996
(general soap-making suppplies, oils)

Cranberry Lane Natural Beauty Products
#65 - 2710 Barnet Hwy
Coquitlam, British Columbia, Canada,
V3B 1B8
(604) 944-1488

Chem Lab Supplies
1060 Ortega Way, Unit C
Placentia, CA 92670
(714) 630-7902
(sodium hydroxide, electronic scales)

Consolidated Plastics Company, Inc.
8181 Darrow Road
Twinsburg, OH 44087
(800) 362-1000
(electronic scales, spatulas,
plastic containers, thermometers)

NOTE *all of the web sites for soap making
also sell oils and fragrances that are used
for making perfumes*

Perfume:

Fragrance Resources
www.fragrance.ch/ www.fragrance.ch

Majestic Mountain Sage
www.the-sage.com/catalog/essential.html

Gingham 'n' Spice
P.O. Box 88psc
Gardenville, PA 18926
(215) 348-3595
(bottles, oils, scented waters)

Cavansons Ltd.
Hollins Vale Works
Hollins Village
Bury, BL9 8QG, UK
(0161) 766-3768

Sunburst Bottle
5710 Auburn Boulevard, Suite #7
Sacramento, CA 95841
(916) 348-5576
(bottles)

General Bottle Supply
P.O. Box 58734
Vernon, CA 90058
(bottles, droppers, lids, glass rods)

Aphrodisia
264 Bleeker Street
New York, NY 10014
(212) 989-6440
(oils, fragrances)

178 soaps & scents

Aromatica
513 N. 36th Street
Seattle, WA 98103
(206) 545-8100
(oils, fragrances)

Garden of Fragrances and Aromatics
141 Court Street
Brooklyn, NY 11201
(718) 625-6340
(oils)

ASSOCIATIONS AND ORGANIZATIONS

International Perfume Bottle Association
www.perfumebottles.org

Perfume Bottle Collecting
members.aol.com/perfumedad/collect2/

Institut Superieur International
du Parfum, de la Cosmetique et de
l'Aromatique Alimentaire
www.isipca.fr

The Fragrance Foundation
www.fragrance.org

The Soap and Detergent Association
www.sdahq.org

The Soap and Detergent Association
475 Park Avenue South
New York, NY 10016
(212) 725-1262

The Fragrance Foundation
145 East 32nd St.
New York, NY 10016
(212) 725-2755

The International Fragrance Association
8 Rue Charles-Humbert
CH-1205 Geneva, Switzerland
011 (41) 22-321-3548

The Cosmetic, Toiletry,
and Fragrance Association
1101 17th Street NW Suite 300
Washington, DC 20036-4702
(202) 331-1770

Le Musée International de la Parfumerie
8, place du Cours
06130 Grasse, France
011 (33) 4- 93-36-80-20

Le Musée du Flacon de Parfum
33, rue du Temple
17000 La Rochelle, France
011 (33) 46 41 32 40.

Aroma and Perfume Museum
Petite Route du Grés-Mas de la Chevêche
Graveson, France
011 (33) 4- 90 95 8152

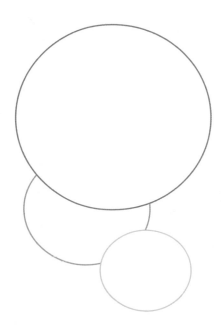

Ackerman, Diane. *A Natural History of the Senses*. Vintage Books, New York, 1991

Bedoukian, Paul Z. *Perfumery and Flavoring Synthetics*. 2nd edition.
    Elsevier Publishing Co., Amsterdam, 1967

Booth, Nancy M. Perfumes, *Splashes & Colognes*. Storey Publishing, Vermont, 1997

Browning, Marie. *Beautiful Handmade Natural Soaps*. Sterling Publishing Co., Inc.
    New York, 1998

Cavitch, Susan Miller. *The Soapmaker's Companion*. Storey Publishing, Vermont,1997

Coss, Melinda. *Le Savon- L'atelier*. Les Editions du Carousel, Paris, 1999

Coney, Norma. *The Complete Soapmaker*. Sterling Publishing Company, Inc.
    New York, 1996

Genders, Roy. *A History of Scent*. Hamish Hamilton Ltd., London, 1972

Green, Annette and Dyett, Lindaq. Secrets of Aromatic Jewelry.
    Flammarion, Paris, 1998

Groom, Nigel. *The Perfume Handbook*. Chapman & Hall, London, 1992

Hulbert, Mike. *Country Living Handmade Soap*. Hearst Books, New York, 1998

Ishaque, Labeena. *Heaven Scent*. Watson-Guptill Publications, New York, 1998

Kaufman, William F. Perfume. *E.P. Dutton & Co.*, Inc., New York, 1974

LaGallienne, Richard. *The Romance of Perfume*. Richard Hudnut, New York, 1928

Lefkowith, Christine Mayer. *The Art of Perfume*. Thames and Hudson Inc.,
    New York, 1994

Maine, Sandy. *The Soap Book: Simple Herbal Recipes*. Interweave Press,
    Colorado, 1995

Mohr, Merilyn. *The Art of Soap Making*. Camden House Publishing, Ontario, 1979

Moran, Jan. *Fabulous Fragrances*. Crescent House Publishing, Beverly Hills, 1994

Newman, Cathy. *Perfume: The Art and Science of Scent*.
National Geographic Society, 1998

Verrill, A. Hyatt. *Perfumes and Spices*.
    L. C. Page & Company Publishers, Boston, 1940

The chart below refers to weights only — never fluid ounces. Be sure to doublecheck your measurements; success in soapmaking relies heavily on accurate amounts.

Ounces	pounds	grams
8 oz	1/2 lb.	226 g
16 oz	1 lb.	454 g
24 oz	1 1/2 lb.	679 g
32 oz	2 lb.	907 g
40 oz	2 1/2 lb.	1.1 kg
48 oz	3 lb.	1.4 kg
56 oz	3 1/2 lb.	1.6 kg
64 oz	4 lb.	1.8 kg
72 oz	4 1/2 lb.	2 kg
80 oz	5 lb.	2.3 kg
88 oz	5 1/2 lb.	2.5 kg
96 oz	6 lb.	2.7 kg

Weight

0.035 ounces	1 gram
1 ounce	28.35 grams
1 pound	453.6 grams

Volume

1 fluid ounce	29.6 mL
1 pint	473 mL
1 quart	946 mL
1 gallon (128 fluid ounces)	3.785

Temperature

To convert Fahrenheit to Celsius: Subtract 32, multiply by 5 and divide by 9.
$100°$ F= (100-32=68; 68x5=340; 340/9=37.8) $37.8°$ C

To convert Celsius to Fahrenheit: Multiply by 9, divide by 5 and add 32.
$37.8°$ C= (37.8x9=340; 340/5=68; 68+32=100) $100°$ F

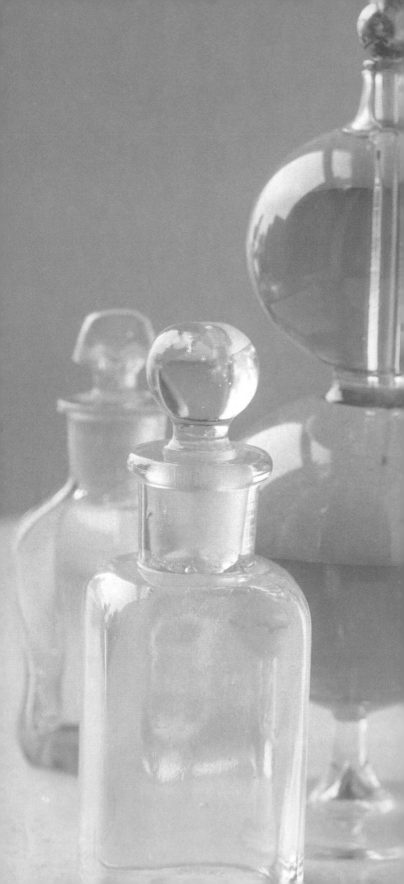

Your Own Custom Blends

You'll discover, as you start to experiment with soaps and perfumes, that it is infinitely useful to keep notes that detail ingredients and dates. Not only will this information help you remember your successful (and not-so-successful) recipes, it will serve as a reminder along the way for important dates in your recipe's aging process. The following is a simple format to help you record this valuable information.

SOAP RECIPE TITLE:

BASIC OILS:

ADDITIVES:

DECORATIVE TOUCHES:

MIXING DATE:
AGING START DATE:
AGING FINISH DATE:

ADDITIONAL NOTES:

SOAP RECIPE TITLE:

BASIC OILS:

ADDITIVES:

DECORATIVE TOUCHES:

MIXING DATE:
AGING START DATE:
AGING FINISH DATE:

ADDITIONAL NOTES:

SOAP RECIPE TITLE:

BASIC OILS:

ADDITIVES:

DECORATIVE TOUCHES:

MIXING DATE:
AGING START DATE:
AGING FINISH DATE:

ADDITIONAL NOTES:

SOAP RECIPE TITLE:

BASIC OILS:

ADDITIVES:

DECORATIVE TOUCHES:

MIXING DATE:
AGING START DATE:
AGING FINISH DATE:

ADDITIONAL NOTES:

SOAP RECIPE TITLE:

BASIC OILS:

ADDITIVES:

DECORATIVE TOUCHES:

MIXING DATE:
AGING START DATE:
AGING FINISH DATE:

ADDITIONAL NOTES:

PERFUME RECIPE TITLE:

BASIC ALCOHOL:

FRAGRANCE & ESSENTIAL OILS:

ADDITIVES:

MIXING DATE:
AGING START DATE:
AGING FINISH DATE:

ADDITIONAL NOTES:

PERFUME RECIPE TITLE:

BASIC ALCOHOL:

FRAGRANCE & ESSENTIAL OILS:

ADDITIVES:

MIXING DATE:
AGING START DATE:
AGING FINISH DATE:

PERFUME RECIPE TITLE:

BASIC ALCOHOL:

FRAGRANCE & ESSENTIAL OILS:

ADDITIVES:

MIXING DATE:
AGING START DATE:
AGING FINISH DATE:

ADDITIONAL NOTES:

PERFUME RECIPE TITLE:

BASIC ALCOHOL:

FRAGRANCE & ESSENTIAL OILS:

ADDITIVES:

MIXING DATE:
AGING START DATE:
AGING FINISH DATE:

ADDITIONAL NOTES:

INDEX